Body Mass Index - Overweight, Normal Weight, Underweight

Edited by Hülya Çakmur

Published in London, United Kingdom

Body Mass Index - Overweight, Normal Weight, Underweight
http://dx.doi.org/10.5772/intechopen.105320
Edited by Hülya Çakmur

Contributors
Teodoro Durá-Travé, Fidel Gallinas-Victoriano, Jitka Kampasová, Hana Válková, Rafik Hadj Aissa, Aissa Bait, Mohamed Guettaf, Fariba Hossein Abadi, Harish Rangareddy, Priyanka Venkatapathappa, Kesava Mandalaneni, Ashakiran Srinivasaiah, Katherine Bourne-Yearwood, Hülya Çakmur, Mahcube Cubukcu, Nur Simsek Yurt

First published in London, United Kingdom, 2023 by IntechOpen
IntechOpen is the global imprint of INTECHOPEN LIMITED, registered in England and Wales, registration number: 11086078, 5 Princes Gate Court, London, SW7 2QJ, United Kingdom

British Library Cataloguing-in-Publication Data
A catalogue record for this book is available from the British Library

Additional hard and PDF copies can be obtained from orders@intechopen.com

Body Mass Index - Overweight, Normal Weight, Underweight
Edited by Hülya Çakmur
p. cm.
Print ISBN 978-1-83768-334-5
Online ISBN 978-1-83768-335-2
eBook (PDF) ISBN 978-1-83768-336-9

For EU product safety concerns:
IN TECH d.o.o., Prolaz Marije Krucifikse Kozulić 3, 51000 Rijeka, Croatia,
info@intechopen.com or visit our website at intechopen.com.

Meet the editor

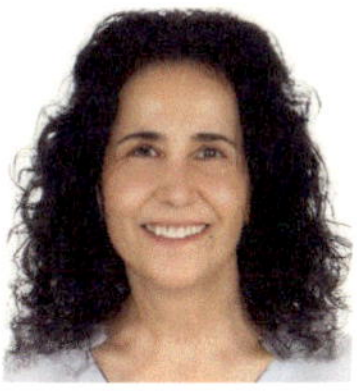

Hülya Çakmur graduated from the medical school at Atatürk University, Turkey. She completed her residency training in family medicine at Trakya University, Turkey. She obtained a Ph.D. in Public Health from Dokuz Eylül University, Turkey. She has 26 years of practice experience as a specialist in family medicine, including 13 years of experience in public health as a Ph.D.-prepared professional. She also studied sleep medicine at the University of Pittsburgh Medical Center, USA, and narrative medicine at St. Thomas University, Canada. She studied voluntarily in geriatrics and published several studies in the field. She is an active member of the Turkish Medical Association and the European Academy of Teachers in General Practice/Family Medicine. She has 12 years of experience as a professor at the University of Kafkas, Turkey, where she is the director of the Department of Family Medicine. She has published more than thirty papers in reputed journals.

Contents

Preface

On the one hand, humanity is trying to cope with diseases caused by hunger and malnutrition and on the other hand, it is struggling with health problems caused by obesity and overweight. It is known that obesity due to all causes (hormonal, genetic, malnutrition, inactivity) is increasing rapidly in all age groups and genders in all developed and developing countries. It is reported that the health problems caused by being underweight are much less than those caused by obesity and overweight. While obesity-related health problems reduce the person's life expectancy and quality on an individual basis, they also harm the economies of countries on a social basis due to workforce loss and health expenses. Alternatively, underweight status is also observed due to some mental disorders (anorexia nervosa, bulimia, etc.) and lack of access to food and malnutrition. All these situations show the importance of maintaining a normal body weight. Body mass index (BMI), which has been in use around the world for nearly a century, is a practical, accessible, and important tool for monitoring the body's normal weight. Although there are various sensitive devices that can measure body fat with full accuracy, BMI will continue to exist for normal weight monitoring due to its easy applicability. This book contains detailed information about BMI (overweight, normal weight and underweight) and various research studies in the field of medicine. For this reason, it is sure to appeal to readers from all segments of society. We would like to thank the authors for their valuable contributions to our book.

With warm regards,

Dr. Hülya Çakmur
Professor,
School of Medicine,
Department of Family Medicine,
Kafkas University,
Kars, Turkey

Chapter 1

Introductory Chapter: A Historical Index Widely Used in Medicine – Body Mass Index

Hülya Çakmur

1. Introduction

Body Mass Index (BMI) which is calculated as a person's weight in kilograms divided by the square of the body height in meters, and is expressed in units of kg/m^2, is still commonly used in the practice of medicine, especially in public health and family medicine, due to its free and easy application [1, 2]. BMI was first defined by Keys and et.al in 1972 and it has not lost its popularity since then [3]. BMI gives a simple numerical result of a person's thinness or thickness thus allowing healthcare professionals to more objectively discuss and monitor weight issues with their patients. For this reason, it seems that it will remain current in medical practice for many years [3, 4].

2. WHO classification of BMI

The World Health Organization (WHO) prescribed BMI and categories to define obesity, overweight, normal weight, and underweight as in below:

Overweight (Pre-obese): 25.0–29.9, Obese (Class I): 30.0–34.9, Obese (Class II): 35.0–39.9, Obese (Class III, Morbid Obese) $\geq$ 40.0, Normal range: 18.5–24.9, Underweight (Mild thinness): 17.0–18.4, Underweight (Moderate thinness): 16.0–16.9, Underweight (Severe thinness): < 16.0 [5].

3. Evaluation of BMI

BMI is a monitoring method, not an exact measurement of the presence and distribution of body fat. There are, of course, individual differences in these evaluation, and BMI is inadequate as the only way to classify a person as obese or malnourished. In certain populations, such as athletes and bodybuilders, high weight as a result of increased muscle mass falsely increases their BMI. For this reason, special regulations should be provided for BMI monitoring [6, 7].

4. Exact way of measuring body fat - bio-electrical impedance

BMI does not directly detect body fat but is as strongly correlated as more direct measures of body fat such as Bio-electrical Impedance Analysis (BIA) which evaluates the body fat makes simultaneous tetrapolar measurements by touching its electrodes [8]. The measurements of the BIA include; lean body mass, skeletal muscle mass, soft tissue mass, total body water amount, intracellular water amount, extracellular water amount, excess body fat, body fat percentage, visceral fat surface, waist-hip ratio, organ fat mass, subcutaneous fat mass, abdominal fat, basal metabolic rate, total energy amount, internal resistance, overweight target control, excess fat target control, and edema parameters and also body mass index. The ideal analysis of the presence and distribution of fat tissue in the human body is, of course, done with such devices [8]. However, these devices are not available everywhere.

5. Healthy body fat and BMI

BMI is one of the tools used to calculate health risks such as physical activity level, smoking, alcohol and substance use, lifestyle, risks of the living environment, blood pressure, cholesterol level, and blood glucose level [2, 3, 9]. Conditions that reduce life expectancy and are associated with mortality, such as overweight, obesity, and diabetes, can also be expected to be associated with high BMI. In addition, it is known that people who are underweight throughout life have a lower premature death rate. However, the optimal BMI at which the risk of death is lowest is unknown [10–12].

6. Obesity and BMI

Obesity, which is chronic systemic inflammation of adipose tissue, when prolonged, eventually activates the innate immune system in adipose tissue. As a result, oxidative stress (OS) increases, which triggers the acute phase response and leads to an inflammatory reaction in the body [13]. Thus, obesity and overweight constitute important risk factors for many acute and chronic diseases, from metabolic and mental diseases to cancer. Obesity not only causes health problems, obesity-related health problems also lead to treatment costs and workforce loss [13, 14]. For this, the presence of fat tissue and its distribution in the body must be evaluated and measured accurately. Excess fat accumulation is usually measured by BMI, which is calculated by weight and height ratios. However, in the presence of abdominal (central) obesity, BMI may appear within normal limits. Therefore, reliable measurement of fat accumulation is necessary, especially in children and the elderly. Healthcare professionals should evaluate BMI while being aware of hidden obesity [15, 16].

The prevalence of obesity is increasing rapidly in every age group and in almost all countries around the world, mostly among low-income and low-educated people. Childhood obesity is a problem that needs to be paid more attention because it is difficult to reverse [13]. In adults, BMI is a useful indicator for assessing health risks throughout life because it is easily calculated and widely available. However, interpreting BMI as an indicator of health risk in children is possible by comparing the child's measurements with age- and gender-specific reference ranges Underestimating the prevalence of obesity, especially in children, as assessed by BMI, may lead to less attention to the problems and inadequate prevention and management. Therefore, a reliable measurement of fat accumulation requires elaborate tools [16].

7. Underweight and BMI

Low body fat, as well as excess body fat, is a risk to body health. People may have low body fat for many different physical (GI disorders, malignancy, infection, thyroid problems, HIV or lung disease, endocrine problems, etc) and mental (such as bulimia, anxiety and stress, dementia, etc.) reasons. In addition to these medical conditions, economic and sociological reasons can also make people underweight because it makes it difficult to access food Detecting and monitoring low body fat ratio is as important as monitoring overweight and obesity. In this case, the most suitable and accessible tool is BMI [11, 17].

8. Limitation of BMI

BMI is an indirect assessment of body fat and therefore already has several deficiencies. Moreover, if it is calculated based on the person's self-reported height and weight, it cannot accurately determine the body fat percentage. For this reason, height and weight measurements must be made by health professionals under optimum conditions and follow-ups must be the same. BMI is a widely used screening tool, but it does not provide clear data on a person's body fat percentage and distribution. As it is known, muscle mass decreases with age. In this case, the shortening of height and decrease in muscle mass with age can be misleading in most cases. Additionally, the relationship between body fat percentage and BMI differs in men and women. For this reason, measurements of waist-hip ratio and skinfold thickness along with BMI lead to more accurate results for body fat ratio [18].

9. Conclusion

BMI is a widely used screening tool to determine body fat percentage. However, it should not be a diagnostic tool. When BMI is to be used due to the lack of a device that accurately measures body fat, these conditions should be taken into consideration in children, the elderly, gender differences, and individuals with excess muscle mass. Although obesity is preventable, it is gradually becoming a pandemic due to the lack of implementation of preventive and sustainable public health approaches. Unfortunately, it is becoming increasingly difficult to acquire and maintain a healthy nutrition culture and life habits. Moreover, naturally obtained nutrients are rapidly decreasing. As obesity continues to increase all over the world, BMI will continue to be used because it is easy to apply.

Author details

Hülya Çakmur
Kafkas University, Turkey

*Address all correspondence to: hulyacakmur@gmail.com

References

[1] Weir CB, Jan A. BMI classification percentile and cut off points. In: StatPearls [Internet]. Treasure Island (FL): StatPearls Publishing; 2023

[2] Gutin I, In BMI. We trust: Reframing the body mass index as a measure of health. Social Theory and Health. 2018;**16**(3):256-271. DOI: 10.1057/s41285-017-0055-0. Epub 2017 Oct 25

[3] Kelly IR, Doytch N, Dave D. How does body mass index affect economic growth? A comparative analysis of countries by levels of economic development. Economics and Human Biology. 2019;**34**:58-73. DOI: 10.1016/j.ehb.2019.03.004. Epub 2019 Mar 11

[4] Chiolero A. Body mass index as socioeconomic indicator. BMJ. 2021;**373**:n1158. DOI: 10.1136/bmj.n1158

[5] A Healthy Lifestyle - WHO Recommendations. 2010. Available from: https://www.who.int/europe/news-room/fact-sheets/item/a-healthy-lifestyle---who-recommendations

[6] Rothman K. BMI-related errors in the measurement of obesity. International Journal of Obesity. 2008;**32**(Suppl 3):S56-S59. DOI: 10.1038/ijo.2008.87

[7] Green DJ. Is body mass index really the best measure of obesity in individuals? Journal of the American College of Cardiology. 2009;**53**(6):526; author reply 527-8. DOI: 10.1016/j.jacc.2008.08.078

[8] Metcalf B, Rabkin RA, Rabkin JM, Metcalf LJ, Lehman-Becker LB. Weight loss composition: The effects of exercise following obesity surgery as measured by bioelectrical impedance analysis. Obesity Surgery. 2005;**15**(2):183-186

[9] Abernathy RP, Black DR. Healthy body weights: An alternative perspective. The American Journal of Clinical Nutrition. 1996;**63**(3 Suppl):448S-451S. DOI: 10.1093/ajcn/63.3.448

[10] Wild SH, Byrne CD. Body mass index and mortality: Understanding the patterns and paradoxes. BMJ. 2016;**353**:i2433. DOI: 10.1136/bmj.i2433

[11] Pepper DJ, Sun J, Suffredini AF, Kadri S. Body-mass index and all-cause mortality. Lancet. 2017;**389**(10086):2284. DOI: 10.1016/S0140-6736(17)31436-8

[12] Friedman GD. Body mass index and risk of death. American Journal of Epidemiology. 2014;**180**(3):233-234. DOI: 10.1093/aje/kwu121. Epub 2014 Jun 3

[13] Wolin KY, Petrelli JM. Obesity. Santa Barbara, CA: Greenwood Press; 2009 ISBN 10: 0313352763/ISBN 13: 9780313352768

[14] Mathus-Vliegen EMH, Basdevant A, Finer N, Hainer V, Hauner H, Micic D, et al. Prevalence, pathophysiology, health consequences and treatment options of obesity in the elderly: A guideline. Obesity Facts. 2012;**5**:460-483. DOI: 10.1159/000341193

[15] Ruderman NB, Schneider SH, Berchtold P. The "metabolically-obese," normal-weight individual. The American Journal of Clinical Nutrition. 1981;**34**(8):1617-1621. DOI: 10.1093/ajcn/34.8.1617

[16] Zemel BS. The challenges of interpreting body mass index in children with obesity. The Journal of Pediatrics. 2021;**235**:21-22. DOI: 10.1016/j.jpeds.2021.04.011. Epub 2021 Apr 13

[17] Lee JY, Kim HC, Kim C, Park K, Ahn SV, Kang DR, et al. Underweight and mortality. Public Health Nutrition. 2016;**19**(10):1751-1756. DOI: 10.1017/S136898001500302X. Epub 2015 Oct 15

[18] Haufs MG, Zöllner YF. Waist-hip ratio more appropriate than body mass index. Deutsches Ärzteblatt International. 2020;**117**(39):659. DOI: 10.3238/arztebl.2020.0659a

Chapter 2

Sexual Dimorphism of the Fat Mass Index and the Fat-Free Mass Index in Healthy Adolescents

Teodoro Durá-Travé and Fidel Gallinas-Victoriano

Abstract

Body mass index (BMI) does not allow to discriminate the composition of the different body compartments. This study points to the formulation of reference values of fat mass index (FMI) and fat-free mass index (FFMI) in healthy adolescents by means of anthropometric techniques, and the subsequent availability in clinical practice as reference charts. The following is a cross-sectional study in a group of 1040 healthy Caucasian adolescents (470 boys and 570 girls), aged 10.1 to 14.9 years. Weight, height and skinfold thickness were registered, and BMI, percentage of total body fat, FMI and FFMI, and FMI and FFMI percentiles were calculated. Boys show a significant increase in FFMI and a decline in body fat and FMI. By contrast, girls show an increase in body fat, FMI and FFMI. Except for the 10 years, FMI was higher ($p < 0.05$) in girls in all ages and FFMI was higher ($p < 0.05$) in boys in all ages. There were no significant differences in the values of BMI between sexes in all ages. The availability of reference values for FMI and FFMI in daily clinical practice would be helpful in the diagnosis and assessment of changes in body composition during the treatment of childhood obesity.

Keywords: adolescents, anthropometric measurements, body composition, body mass index, fat mass index, fat-free mass index, skinfold thickness

1. Introduction

The percentage of children categorized as overweight and obesity in children has increased firmly, to the extent that it has become the most relevant nutritional disorder in present-day developed society [1]. In this way, this percentage of excess body weight in otherwise healthy adolescents in our community (Navarra, Spain) hits 22.5% [2]. This figure is comparable to the values in other regions of our country (Spain), the European countries, and the USA, and it even exceeds the eastern European countries [1, 3].

Obesity implies an excess of body fat, and the most adequate and usual anthropometric measure for the initial nutritional assessment in clinical practice is the body mass index (BMI) [4]. Despite this potential in the diagnosis of obesity, this parameter does not define the percent distribution of the body compartments (fat mass and fat-free mass). As a matter of fact, different studies promote FMI before the BMI in the diagnosis and assessment of childhood obesity, claiming a higher sensibility in the detection of changes in body fat [5–8].

Notwithstanding the above, FMI is not satisfactorily extended in the diagnosis and assessment of childhood obesity and, consequently, few referent charts for pediatricians are available at the present day [9, 10]. The evaluation by means of anthropometric measures, as a consequence of the relative simplicity and low cost, is regarded as an important stage in the evaluation of body composition at the pediatric age and should have a primary role in the assessment process [6, 10–14]. In fact, the accessibility to FMI and FFMI reference charts based on the measures of body skin folds would largely help in the evaluation.

The aim of the present work is to compile standard values charts for FMI and FFMI in healthy adolescents (both sexes), from the measurement of skin folds in order to be available as benchmarks in daily clinical practice.

2. Methods

2.1 Participants

The design of the study was cross-sectional and the sample consisted of 1040 individuals (470 boys and 570 girls). All of them were Caucasian adolescents, aged 10.1 to 14.9 years, students of the different corresponding grades of four public schools located in Pamplona (Navarre, Spain) and enrolled specifically for this survey. The period of study was January–June 2018.

Pamplona is a city located in the north region of Spain, with a population of 203 382 inhabitants (2018 census, Instituto de Estadística de Navarra). The population corresponding to the range 10.1 to 14.9 years is 9772 (4.8% of the total population) in the year 2018, distributed as 5042 boys and 4680 girls. The calculation of the sample size was made assuming the worst-case estimate (0.50), with a 95% confidence level and a precision of 0.04, thereby resulting in a number of 600 participants as the minimum required.

All legal guardians/parents had plenty information of about the survey and written consent available in order to participate in this study.

A normal nutrition study was a mandatory condition in order to be included in this study: BMI value should be in the range +1/ −1 SD. Other causes of exclusion were non-Caucasian origin and previous chronic pathologies that may influence growth, body composition, food ingestion, or physical activity.

An informed consent was provided to 1451 legal guardians (763 boys and 740 girls). From the initial 763 boys, 62 individuals did not add the consent in time or had some failure in the completion, 136 individuals suffered from excess weight (overweight/obesity, BMI> 1SD), 78 individuals were excluded because of ethnic reasons (non-Caucasian family origin), and 17 individuals did not meet the preconditions (chronic pathologies, etc.). Subsequently, the number of remaining participants was 470. Of the initial 740 girls, 49 did not complete adequately the consent, 53 presented with excess weight (overweight/obesity BMI>1 SD), 57 because of ethnic origin (non-Caucasian), and 11 because of other preconditions (chronic pathologies, etc.). Therefore, the total of recruited girls was 570. In this way, the response rate after the appropriate disposal was 92.1%, and the total response rate in both sexes was 90.4.

This study meets with the terms and conditions of the local Ethics Committee for Human investigation (Navarre University Hospital) in accordance with the ethical standards established by the 1964 Declaration of Helsinki and posterior amendments.

2.2 Anthropometric measurements

Different anthropometric measures were recorded during clinical evaluation at the consultation: height, weight, body mass index, (BMI), and skinfold thickness (in the different localizations: biceps, triceps, subscapular, and suprailiac regions).

A clinical examination with the patient in underclothes and barefoot was completed. The measurement of weight required an Año-Savol scale (reading interval 0 to 120 kg and precision of 100 g) and the measurement of height was made with a Holtain wall stadiometer (reading interval 60 to 120 cm, precision 0.1 cm). These measures allowed subsequent calculation of BMI by means of the corresponding formula: weight (kg)/height^2 (m).

Three consecutive skinfold-thickness measurements were recorded in the corresponding anatomical locations: the biceps (front side middle upper arm), the triceps (back side middle upper arm), subscapular (right beneath the lowest point of the scapula), and suprailiac (right above the iliac crest of the hip bone). All of them were performed by the same-trained person and the average of the three measures was the figure to be used in the estimate. The skinfold values were taken with a precision of 0.1 mm on the left side of the body with the Holtain skinfold caliper (CMS Weighing Equipment, Crymych, United Kingdom). The calculation of the percentage of total body fat, fat mass (kg) and fat-free mass (kg) required the use of the formulas delivered by Slaughter et al. [15], adjusted for sex and age. Additionally, the FMI and the FFMI were estimated with the formulas: fat mass (kg)/height^2 (m), and free fat mass (kg)/height^2 (m), respectively.

Secondarily, the z-score values for the BMI were calculated with the Aplicación Nutricional, from the Spanish Society of pediatric gastroenterology, hepatology, and nutrition (available at http://www.gastroinf.es/nutritional/). The graphics from Ferrández et al. (Centro Andrea Prader, Zaragoza 2002) were used as reference charts [16].

2.3 Statistical analysis

The program Statistical Packages for the Social Sciences version 20.0 (SPSS, Chicago, IL, USA) was used to perform the statistical analysis (descriptive statistics, percentiles calculation, Student's t test, and analysis of variance), and the results are shown as means (M) and standard deviations (SD). The condition for statistical significance was a p-value <0.05.

3. Results

Table 1 illustrates the values and the comparison of the different anthropometric measurements and the estimation of body composition according to age in adolescent boys. As can be noted, a significant increase in the mean values of weight, height, BMI, fat mass, fat-free mass, and FFMI is discernible ($p < 0.05$). On the contrary, the comparison of the mean values of body fat, skinfold thickness (triceps), and FMI reveal a significant decrease ($p < 0.05$). No significant differences were found

	10 y ($n = 82$)	11 y ($n = 84$)	12 y ($n = 112$)	13 y ($n = 108$)	14 y ($n = 84$)	p-value*
Age (y)	10.4 ± 0.3	11.5 ± 0.2	12.4 ± 0.2	13.4 ± 0.2	14.2 ± .1	0.001
Weight (kg)	37.9 ± 6.1	39.8 ± 5.5	43.2 ± 7.6	49.3 ± 7.8	54.1 ± 9.1	0.001
Height (cm)	142.0 ± 9.7	146.5 ± 8.2	153.4 ± 9.5	158.7 ± 9.6	164.8 ± 9.4	0.001
BMI (kg/m^2)	18.7 ± 1.5	18.9 ± 1.5	19.2 ± 1.5	19.6 ± 1.6	20.3 ± 1.7	0.001
BMI z-score	0.08 ± 0.61	0.02 ± 0.56	0.01 ± 0.54	0.05 ± 0.57	0.05 ± 0.05	0.072
Skinfold thickness						
Biceps (mm)	9.1 ± 3.5	8.9 ± 2.9	9.1 ± 3.8	8.3 ± 4.2	8.9 ± 4.1	0.508
Triceps (mm)	14.2 ± 3.7	14.5 ± 4.1	13.9 ± 5.1	13.4 ± 5.2	13.5 ± 4.9	0.028
Subscapular (mm)	9.9 ± 4.1	9.8 ± 4.3	10.3 ± 5.1	10.2 ± 5.3	10.2 ± 3.9	0.222
Suprailiac (mm)	12.3 ± 6.3	12.4 ± 6.5	12.2 ± 6.1	12.6 ± 6.8	12.4 ± 6.4	0.328
Body fat (%)	25.4 ± 5.8	24.4 ± 4.5	23.1 ± 5.9	21.5 ± 5.9	22.4 ± 5.9	0.001
Fat mass (kg)	9.7 ± 3.1	9.7 ± 2.9	10.1 ± 3.8	10.2 ± 3.7	11.9 ± 4.1	0.001
Fat-free mass (kg)	28.2 ± 4.3	28.7 ± 4.1	32.7 ± 5.6	37.1 ± 5.8	39.8 ± 6.1	0.001
FMI (kg/m^2)	4.8 ± 1.4	4.6 ± 1.2	4.4 ± 1.4	4.2 ± 1.4	4.3 ± 1.5	0.003
FFMI (kg/m^2)	13.8 ± 0.7	14.2 ± 0.9	14.7 ± 0.9	15.3 ± 0.9	15.6 ± 0.7	0.001

**ANOVA. BMI, body mass index; FMI, fat mass index; FFMI, fat-free mass index.*

Table 1.
Anthropometric measurements and body composition in adolescent boys (M ± SD).

Age	p3	p10	p25	p50	p75	p90	p97
Fat mass index (kg/m^2)							
10 y	2.78	2.85	3.79	4.29	6.25	7.32	7.45
11 y	2.47	2.86	3.58	4.22	5.91	6.93	7.45
12 y	2.17	2.90	3.38	4.15	5.57	6.54	7.46
13 y	2.15	2.48	3.09	4.10	5.56	6.52	6.81
14 y	2.21	2.38	3.07	4.61	5.82	6.76	6.95
Fat-free mass index (kg/m^2)							
10 y	12.25	12.90	13.45	13.93	14.28	14.8	15.12
11 y	12.75	13.10	13.74	14.39	14.86	15.57	15.85
12 y	13.28	13.33	13.96	14.84	15.41	16.35	16.61
13 y	13.38	14.27	14.61	15.32	15.81	17.11	17.85
14 y	14.35	14.81	15.31	15.51	16.17	16.91	17.44

p, percentile.

Table 2.
Percentiles values for fat mass index and fat-free mass index in adolescent boys in different ages.

in the comparison of the mean values of BMI z-score and skinfold thickness (biceps, subscapular, and suprailiac).

Table 2 displays the percentile distribution corresponding to FFMI and FMI in adolescent boys according to age.

Table 3 shows the mean values and the comparison of the anthropometric measurements and the estimation of body composition according to age in adolescent girls. A significant increase ($p < 0.05$) in the mean values of weight, height, BMI, skinfold thickness (subscapular and suprailiac), body fat, fat mass, fat-free mass, FMI, and FFMI can be appreciated. The comparison of the mean values of BMI z-score and skinfold thickness (biceps and triceps) showed no significant differences.

Table 4 lists the percentile distribution of FFMI and FMI in adolescent girls according to age.

Figure 1 presents the comparison of the mean values of FMI in both sexes for the different ages. Excluding the period 10–11 years, a significant increase ($p < 0.05$) in the values of FMI is detected in girls with respect to boys in the different age groups.

Figure 2 displays the values of FFMI in both sexes in the different ages and compares them. Significantly higher ($p < 0.05$) values are recorded in boys of all ages.

There were no significant differences in the values of BMI between sexes in all ages (**Figure 3**).

	10 y ($n = 148$)	11 y ($n = 108$)	12 y ($n = 110$)	13 y ($n = 104$)	14 y ($n = 100$)	p-value*
Age (y)	10.4 ± 0.2	11.5 ± 0.3	12.4 ± 0.3	13.4 ± .2	14.3 ± 0.2	0.001
Weight (kg)	38.1 ± 5.3	42.8 ± 6.4	46.0 ± 6.7	49 ± 6.9	52.2 ± 8.1	0.001
Height (cm)	143.0 ± 7.3	149 ± 8.6	154.1 ± 8.5	157.7 ± 8.2	159.8 ± 7.1	0.001
BMI (kg/m^2)	18.6 ± 1.4	19.3 ± 1.6	19.7 ± 1.9	20.1 ± 1.7	20.8 ± 1.9	0.001
BMI z-score	0.09 ± 0.5	0.09 ± 0.53	0.04 ± 0.64	0.05 ± 0.57	0.02 ± 0.67	0.086
Skinfold thickness						
Biceps (mm)	10.3 ± 3.4	10.3 ± 3.9	10.1 ± 2.8	10.4 ± 3.3	10.9 ± 3.2	0.709
Triceps (mm)	16.1 ± 3.9	15.8 ± 4.4	15.9 ± 4.4	16.3 ± 4.5	16.9 ± 3.7	0.738
Subscapular (mm)	10.9 ± 4.2	11.4 ± 4.8	11.1 ± 4.1	12.2 ± 5.2	13.1 ± 5.1	0.002
Suprailiac (mm)	14.4 ± 6.1	15.7 ± 6.5	15.9 ± 6.5	17.7 ± 7.1	18.2 ± 6.4	0.001
Body fat (%)	27.4 ± 5.9	28.3 ± 4.3	28.6 ± 3.7	29.2 ± 4.2	29.3 ± 3.5	0.005
Fat mass (kg)	10.7+3.3	12.5 ± 3.0	13.0 ± 3.1	14.3 ± 2.8	15.6 ± 3.8	0.001
Fat-free mass (kg)	27.7 ± 3.2	31.3 ± 4.4	33.7 ± 4.4	34.7 ± 4.3	37.0 ± 4.4	0.001
FMI (kg/m^2)	5.1 ± 1.4	5.5 ± 1.2	5.7 ± 1.1	5.9 ± 1.2	6.2 ± 1.2	0.001
FFMI (kg/m^2)	13.4 ± 0.8	13.8 ± 0.8	14.2 ± 0.9	14.3 ± 0.9	14.7 ± 0.9	0.001

**ANOVA. BMI, body mass index; FMI, fat mass index; FFMI, fat-free mass index.*

Table 3.
Anthropometric measurements and body composition in adolescent girls (M ± SD).

Age	p 3	p 10	p 25	p 50	p 75	p 90	p 97
Fat mass index (kg/m^2)							
10 y	2.79	3.46	3.92	5.33	6.24	7.31	7.74
11 y	3.57	3.77	4.68	5.49	6.30	7.21	7.89
12 y	3.75	4.12	4.68	5.18	6.40	7.33	7.88
13 y	3.89	3.99	4.83	5.91	7.07	7.79	7.90
14 y	4.08	4.80	5.02	6.46	6.99	8.28	8.60
Fat-free mass index (kg/m^2)							
10 y	12.05	12.31	12.84	13.54	14.04	14.53	14.91
11 y	12.48	12.79	13.17	13.87	14.39	14.86	15.52
12 y	12.86	13.04	13.54	14.29	15.07	15.76	16.31
13 y	12.77	12.78	13.62	14.21	14.45	16.12	16.35
14 y	12.84	13.00	13.87	14.88	15.61	16.00	16.55

p, percentile.

Table 4.
Percentiles values for fat mass index and fat-free mass index in adolescent girls in different ages.

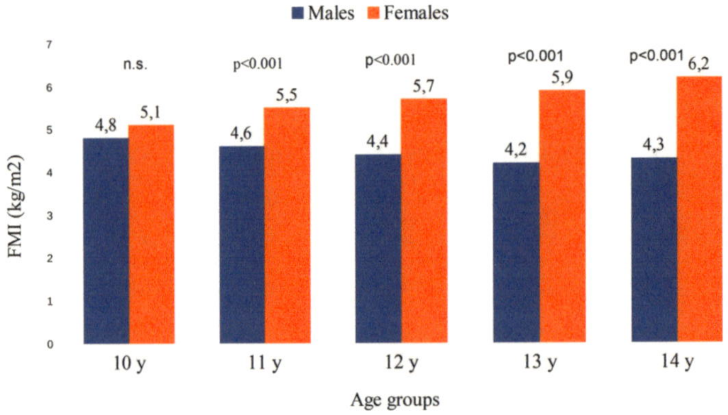

Figure 1.
Gender differences for FMI in each of the ages.

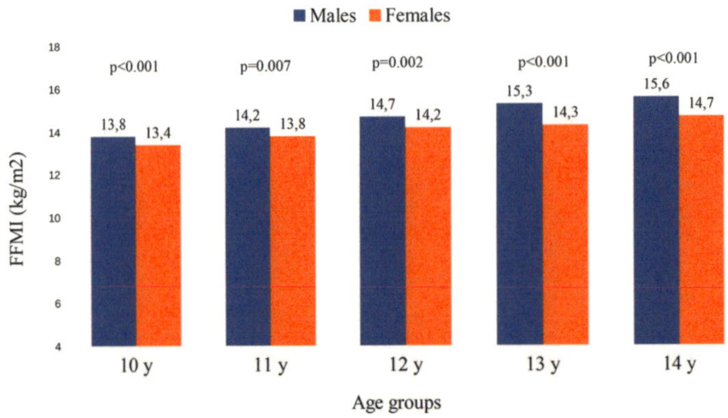

Figure 2.
Gender differences for FFMI in each of the ages.

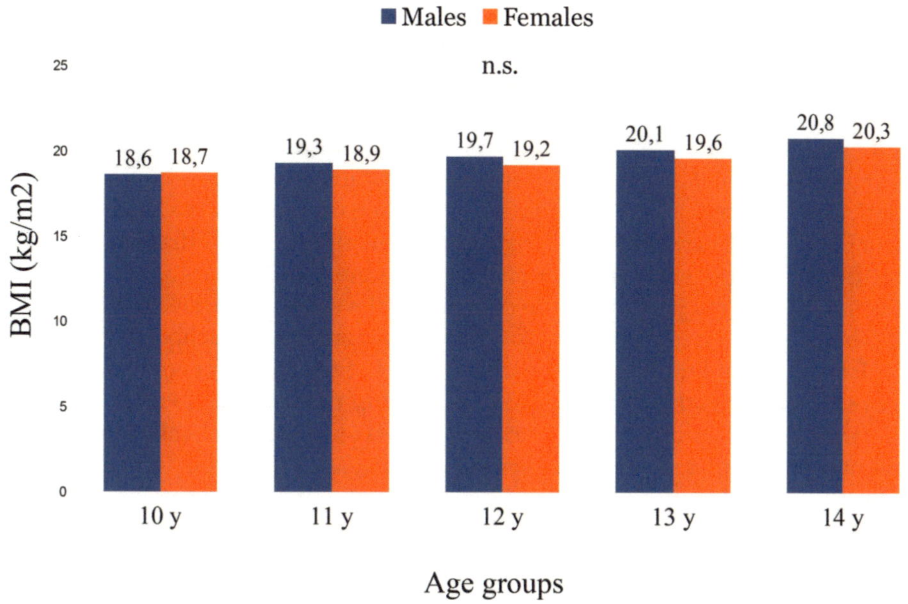

Figure 3.
Gender differences for BMI in each of the ages.

4. Discussion

The analysis of the different measurements and the changes in the estimation of the body compartments (fat mass and fat-free mass) in adolescents (range 10–14 years) with normal BMI values adjusted for age and sex shows a different pattern depending on sex. The FFMI shows a progressive and significant increase in both sexes related to age, but boys present with significantly higher values than girls do. Additionally, FMI decreases progressively and significantly in boys in relation to age, in comparison with the progressive and significant increase observed in girls. It should be noted that these changes occur concurrently with a continuous increase in BMI in both sexes in these life stages in the absence of significant differences in BMI values in both sexes.

The nutrition status classification of the participants in this study was established on the basis of the results the BMI. This index has proved to be useful in the definition of overweight and obesity [4, 6, 17, 18], but it provides limited information because it implies excessive weight in relation to height rather than excess body fat. In other words, the relative composition of the body compartments (fat mass and fat-free mass) is not adequately determined [19–23]. Furthermore, this limitation is even more marked during adolescence, a period of life in which several physical and physiological changes take place [24, 25], and weight gain does not necessarily imply excessive fat accumulation [26, 27]. In this way, the availability of a list of FMI and FFMI standardized values for healthy adolescents enables to differentiate between individuals that show high BMI values and, simultaneously, present with low FFMI and high FMI values (a condition that matches the criteria of overweight or obesity), and those that also show high BMI values and, simultaneously, present with high FFMI and low FMI (a condition that corresponds rather to muscle hypertrophy, and is reasonably frequent in adolescent boys).

The availability of reference charts for FMI and FFMI in the pediatric age is limited, and they require sophisticated methodologies, what makes them difficult to access in clinical practice, such as dual-energy X-ray absorptiometry or isotope dilution [9, 10, 28]; that is, the reason why they are used primarily in the investigation. Nonetheless, it has been corroborated that the values delivered with anthropometric measurements are in close correlation with those obtained with these high-cost and sophisticated techniques [6, 10–14, 29, 30]; even the easier models that divide the body in FM and FFM are as applicable as the more complex models that separate FFM in its different components (water, minerals, and proteins) [28].

The selection of the participants in the study is the main limitation we encountered. They were selected from the most crowded centers (public schools) of the city of Pamplona, and therefore the marginal zones of the city were not included. Moreover, students from private schools did not enter the study, and variables that could condition the results, like socioeconomic level or parental schooling and education were not included either. Even so, the participant eligibility criteria that were proposed for this study (BMI between +1 and −1 SD) allowed passing over these potential differences. All participants were healthy and showed BMI values in range, and so a typical and progressive pubertal development was assumed, being this condition a potential limitation. This assumption is reasonable and, in point of fact, basically every chart of anthropometric variables (height, weight, BMI, etc.), either cross-sectional of longitudinal, that is used in clinical practice refers entirely to the chronological age of the individuals [16, 31–35].

The precision of the measurements of skinfold thickness has been contested because of the hypothetical operator dependency. According to our experience, and in line with other authors, the FMI (evaluated by skin folds) can be used as a valid predictor of the changes in body fat composition in childhood obesity [6, 17, 36]. Bioelectrical impedance analysis (BIA) is an alternative approach in the evaluation of body composition through the measurement of impedance or resistance and reactance values of a small electric current as it spreads through the body water. BIA is a low-cost and noninvasive technique with high reproducibility, easy usage of the equipment, and low operator dependency. The majority of studies based on BIA have been undertaken in the adult population, they demand methodological or standardization rules in order to perform measurements in children, especially concerning fasting, hydration, voiding, clothing, skin preparation, and body position [37]. Furthermore, BIA might underestimate fat mass and overestimate fat-free mass in healthy as well as obese children [38–40], perhaps in relation to these methodological issues. In other words, BIA can be considered a valuable method, but we need additional studies focused on methodological issues to provide definitive guidelines for the standardization of these measurements in the child population.

5. Conclusion

The availability of valid charts (based on the measurements of skin thickness) for the application as reference patterns in healthy adolescents of both sexes in clinical practice would be very helpful for the diagnosis and, particularly, the analysis of the changes in body composition that occur during the treatment of childhood obesity. In fact, more studies are required to provide support the conclusions of the analysis of these data, as well as to evaluate its usefulness in clinical practice.

Funding

The authors received no financial support for the research, authorship, and/or publication of this article.

Conflict of interest

The authors declared no potential conflicts of interest with respect to the research, authorship, and/or publication of this study.

Author details

Teodoro Durá-Travé[1,2,3]* and Fidel Gallinas-Victoriano[2,3]

1 Department of Pediatrics, School of Medicine, University of Navarra, Pamplona, Spain

2 Department of Pediatrics, Navarra University Hospital, Pamplona, Spain

3 Navarrabiomed (Biomedical Research Center), Pamplona, Spain

*Address all correspondence to: tdura@unav.es

References

[1] Lissau I, Overpeck MD, Ruan WJ, Due P, Holstein HML. Body mass index and overweight in adolescents in 13 European countries, Israel, and the United States. Archives of Pediatrics & Adolescent Medicine. 2004;**158**:27-33

[2] Durá-Travé T, Hualde-Olascoaga J, Garralda-Torres I. Overweight among children in Navarra (Spain) and its impact on adolescence. Medicina Clínica (Barcelona). 2012;**138**:52-56

[3] Knai C, Suhrcke M, Lobstein T. Obesity in Eastern Europe: An overview of its health and economic implications. Economics and Human Biology. 2007;**5**:392-408

[4] Styne DM, Arslanian SA, Connor EL, Farooqi IS, Murad MH, Silverstein JH, et al. Pediatric obesity-assessment, treatment, and prevention: An endocrine society clinical practice guideline. The Journal of Clinical Endocrinology and Metabolism. 2017;**102**:709-757

[5] Schutz Y, Kyle UU, Pichard C. Fat-free mass index and fat mass index percentiles in Caucasians aged 18-98 y. International Journal of Obesity and Related Metabolic Disorders. 2002;**26**:953-960

[6] De Miguel-Etayo P, Moreno LA, Santabarbara J, Martín-Matillas M, Piqueras MJ, Rocha-Silva D, et al. Anthropometric indices to assess body-fat changes during a multidisciplinary obesity treatment in adolescents: EVASYON Study. Clinical Nutrition. 2015;**34**:523-528

[7] Okorodudu DO, Jumean MF, MontoriVM,Romero-CorralA,SomersVK, Erwin PJ, et al. Diagnostic performance of body mass index to identify obesity as defined by body adiposity: A systematic review and meta-analysis. International Journal of Obesity. 2010;**34**:791-799

[8] Pereira-da-Silva L, Dias MP, Dionísio E, Virella D, Alves M, Diamantino C, et al. Fat mass index performs best in monitoring management of obesity in prepubertal children. Jornal de Pediatria. 2016;**92**(4):421-426

[9] Nakao T, Komiya S. Reference norms for a fat-free mass index and fat mass index in the Japanese child population. Journal of Physiological Anthropology and Applied Human Science. 2003;**22**:293-298

[10] Wells JC, Williams JE, Chomtho S, Darch T, Grijalva-Eternod C, Kennedy K, et al. Body composition reference data for simple and reference techniques and a 4-component model: A new UK reference child. The American Journal of Clinical Nutrition. 2012;**96**:1316-1326

[11] Weyers AM, Mazzetti SA, Love DM, Gomez AL, Kraemer WJ, Volek JS. Comparison of methods for assessing body composition changes during weight loss. Medicine and Science in Sports and Exercise. 2002;**34**:497-502

[12] Elberg J, McDuffie JR, Sebring NG, Salaita C, Keil M, Robotham D, et al. Comparison of methods to assess change in children's body com-position. The American Journal of Clinical Nutrition. 2004;**80**:64-69

[13] Sopher AB, Thornton JC, Wang J, Pierson RN, Heymsfield SB, Horlick M. Measurement of percentage of body fat in 411 children and adolescents: A comparison of dual-energy X-ray absorptiometry with a four-compartment model. Pediatrics. 2004;**113**:1285-1290

[14] Martin-Calvo N, Moreno-Galarraga L, Martinez-Gonzalez MA. Association between body mass index, waist-to-height ratio and adiposity in children: A systematic review and meta-analysis. Nutrients. 2016;**8**(8):512

[15] Slaughter MH, Lohman TG, Boileau RA, Horswill CA, Stillman RJ, van Loan MD, et al. Skinfold equations for estimation of body fatness in children and youths. Human Biology. 1988;**60**:709-723

[16] Ferrandez A, Baguer L, Labarta JL, Labena C, Mayayo E, Puba B. Longitudinal pubertal growth according to age at pubertal study of normal Spanish children from birth to adulthood. Pediatric Endocrinology Reviews. 2005;**2**:423-559

[17] Durá-Travé T, Gallinas-Victoriano F, Urretavizcaya-Martinez M, Ahmed-Mohamed L, Guindulain MJC, Berrade-Zubiri S. Assessment of body composition changes during a combined intervention for the treatment of childhood obesity. Nutrition. 2019;**59**:116-120

[18] Alves CAS, Mocellin MC, Andrade-Gonçalves EC, Silva DAS, Trindade EBSM. Anthropometric Indicators as Body Fat Discriminators in Children and Adolescents: A Systematic Review and Meta-Analysis. Advances in Nutrition. 2017;**8**:718-727

[19] Freedman DS, Wang J, Thornton JC, Mei Z, Sopher AB, Pierson RN, et al. Classification of body fatness by body mass index-for-age categories among children. Archives of Pediatrics & Adolescent Medicine. 2009;**163**:805-811

[20] Javed A, Jumean M, Murad MH, Okorodudu D, Kumar S, Somers VK, et al. Diagnostic performance of body mass index to identify obesity as defined by body adiposity in children and adolescents: A systematic review and meta-analysis. Pediatric Obesity. 2015;**10**:234-244

[21] Mei Z, Grummer-Strawn LM, Pietrobelli A, Goulding A, Goran MI, Dietz WH. Validity of body mass index compared with other body-composition screening indexes for the assessment of body fatness in children and adolescents. The American Journal of Clinical Nutrition. 2002;**75**:978-985

[22] Frankenfield DC, Rowe WA, Cooney RN, Smith JS, Becker D. Limits of body mass index to detect obesity and predict body composition. Nutrition. 2001;**17**:26-30

[23] Demerath EW, Schubert CM, Maynard LM, Sun SS, Chumlea WC, Pickoff A, et al. Do changes in body mass index percentile reflect changes in body composition in children? Data from the Fels Longitudinal Study. Pediatrics. 2006;**117**:e487-e495

[24] Odgen CL, Li Y, Freedman DS, Borrud LG, Flegal KM. Smoothed percentage body fat percentiles for U.S. children and adolescents, 1999-2004. National Health Statistics Reports. 2011;**9**:1-7

[25] Kurtoglu S, Mazicioglu MM, Ozturk A, Hatipoglu N, Cicek B, Ustunbas HB. Body fat reference curves for healthy Turkish children and adolescents. European Journal of Pediatrics. 2010;**169**:1329-1335

[26] Eissa MA, Dai S, Mihalopoulos NL, Day RS, Harrist RB, Labarthe DR. Trajectories of fat mass index, fat free-mass index, and waist circumference in children: Project HeartBeat! American Journal of Preventive Medicine. 2009;**37**(Suppl. 1):S34-S39

[27] Hattori K, Tahara Y, Moji K, Aoyagi K, Furusawa T. Chart analysis of body composition change among pre- and postadolescent Japanese subjects assessed by underwater weighing method. International Journal of Obesity and Related Metabolic Disorders. 2004;**28**:520-524

[28] Vasquez F, Salazar G, Diaz E, Lera L, Anziani A, Burrows R. Comparison of body fat calculations by sex and puberty status in obese schoolchildren using two and four compartment body composition models. Nutrición Hospitalaria. 2016;**33**:1116-1122

[29] Rodríguez G, Moreno LA, Blay MG, Blay VA, Fleta J, Sarría A, et al. Body fat measurement in adolescents: Comparison of skinfold thickness equations with dual-energy X-ray absorptiometry. European Journal of Clinical Nutrition. 2005;**59**:1158-1166

[30] Martín-Matillas M, Mora-Gonzalez J, Migueles JH, Ubago-Guisado E, Gracia-Marco L, Ortega FB. Validity of slaughter equations and bioelectrical impedance against dual-energy X-ray absorptiometry in children. Obesity (Silver Spring). 2020;**28**:803-812

[31] Wright CM, Booth IW, Buckler JM, Cameron N, Cole TJ, Healy MJ, et al. Growth reference charts for use in the United Kingdom. Archives of Disease in Childhood. 2002;**86**:11-14

[32] Deheeger M, Rolland-Cachera MF. Etude longitudinales de la croissance d'enfants parisiens suivis de l'age de 10 mois a 18 ans. Archives de Pédiatrie. 2004;**11**:1130-1144

[33] Durá-Travé T, Garralda-Torres I, Hualde-Olascoaga J. Longitudinal study of child growth in Navarre (1993-2007). Anales de Pediatría (Barcelona, Spain). 2009;**70**:526-533

[34] The 2000 CDC Growth Charts. Clinical Growth Charts. Available from http://www.cdc.gov/growthcharts/clinical_charts.htm

[35] WHO Child growth standards growth reference data for 5-19 years. Available from http://www.who.int/growthref/en/

[36] Durá-Travé G-VF, Urretavizacaya-Martinez M, Ahmed-Mohamed L, Chueca-Guindulain MJ, Berrade-Zubiri S. Effects of the application of a prolonged combined intervention on body composition in adolescents with obesity. Nutrition Journal. 2020;**19**:49

[37] Brantlov S, Ward LC, Jodal L, Ritting S, Lange A. Critical factors and their impact on bioelectrical impedance analysis in children: A review. Journal of Medical Engineering & Technology. 2017;**41**:22-35

[38] Kyle UG, Earthman CP, Pichard C, Coss-Bu JA. Body composition during growth in children: Limitations and perspectives of bioelectrical impedance analysis. European Journal of Clinical Nutrition. 2015;**69**:1298-1305

[39] Chula de Castro JA, Rodrigues de Lima T, Santos-Silva DA. Body composition estimation in children and adolescents by bioelectrical impedance analysis: A systematic review. Journal of Bodywork and Movement Therapies. 2018;**22**:134-136

[40] Seo Y, Kim JH, Kim Y, Lim H, Ju Y, Kang MJ, et al. Validation of body composition using bioelectrical impedance analysis in children according to the degree of obesity. Scandinavian Journal of Medicine & Science in Sports. 2018;**28**:2207-2215

Chapter 3

Leptin and Obesity: Understanding the Impact on Dyslipidemia

Harish Rangareddy, Priyanka Venkatapathappa, Kesava Mandalaneni, Ashakiran Srinivasaiah and Katherine Bourne-Yearwood

Abstract

Leptin, a hormone produced by fat cells, regulates energy balance and body weight by suppressing appetite and increasing energy expenditure. In obesity, there is often leptin resistance, reducing the hormone's effects due to factors such as inflammation and changes in leptin receptors. This resistance leads to an increased risk of weight gain and obesity. Leptin therapy shows promise in treating obesity and related metabolic disorders, such as dyslipidemia and type 2 diabetes mellitus. It can lower body weight, improve insulin sensitivity, and reduce blood glucose and lipid levels. However, its effectiveness may be limited by the development of leptin resistance. Leptin also exhibits anti-inflammatory and cardiovascular protective effects, with potential therapeutic value for obesity-related conditions. Nevertheless, further research is necessary to comprehend leptin's mechanisms and develop safe and effective therapies for these conditions, including those targeting dyslipidemia.

Keywords: adipokines, leptin receptors, obesity, lipid metabolism, atherosclerosis

1. Introduction

Obesity, which is characterized by excessive body fat accumulation, is a major contributor to dyslipidemia. Leptin, a hormone secreted by adipose tissue, plays a crucial role in regulating energy balance, including appetite and metabolism.

Leptin resistance, a condition where the body is insensitive to leptin, is common in obesity, and it may contribute to dyslipidemia by altering lipid metabolism and promoting inflammation. Understanding the complex interplay between leptin, obesity, and dyslipidemia is crucial for developing effective strategies for the prevention and treatment of CVD. By elucidating the underlying mechanisms and pathways involved, researchers and clinicians can identify potential targets for intervention and develop personalized treatment plans for individuals with dyslipidemia and obesity.

1.1 Overview of obesity as a global epidemic

Obesity is a pandemic with potentially fatal effects on human health. Within the last 20 years, the prevalence of this condition has tripled globally, and it is still rising [1].

Studies have shown that obesity is influenced by genetics. It appears to be a polygenic condition based on the inheritance pattern, with minor contributions from several distinct genes, accounting for almost 25–70% of the variance in weight [2]. A BMI of >30 kg/m^2 is measured as obese per the International Obesity Task Force and the WHO categorization [3]. The illness causes several systemic problems. The distribution of fat, rather than the total quantity of extra adipose tissue, appears to be significant for some of the consequences of obesity [4]. Additionally, obesity negatively impacts morbidity and death [5]. As its growing prevalence and importance are undeniable in today's context, it would be worthwhile to discuss the various aspects of this disease.

Obesity is a medical condition characterized by an excessive accumulation of body fat that can have negative effects on health, including a shortened lifespan and increased health problems. It is classified as having a body weight that is at least 20% above the usual range. Overweight (pre-obesity) is defined as having a body mass index (BMI), which compares weight to height, between 25 and 30 kg/m^2, while obesity is defined as having a BMI greater than 30 kg/m^2. Overweight and obesity are characterized by abnormal or excessive deposits of fat that pose health risks. Hyperplastic obesity refers to an increase in the number of fat cells, while hypertrophic obesity refers to an increase in the size of fat cells, or a combination of both [1].

BMI is a statistical evaluation based on height and weight. The proportion of body fat is not measured, although it is thought to be beneficial for estimating healthy body weight. The BMI measurement can occasionally be deceiving; for example, a muscleman may have a high BMI yet have far less body fat than an unhealthy individual with a lower BMI. BMI serves as a useful indicator for the "typical person" in general. Body mass index, equal to weight in kg/height in m^2, is the most often used measurement to assess obesity, despite not being a direct indicator of adiposity [6].

Classification of adults according to BMI:

1. Underweight<18.5

2. Normal range: 18.5–24.99

3. Overweight: >25

    a. Pre obese: 25–29.99

    b. Obese Class I: 30–34.99

    c. Obese II: 35–39.99

    d. Obese III: >40 [6]

Anthropometry (measures the thickness of skin folds), hydrodensitometry (underwater weighing), CT or MRI, and electrical impedance are additional methods for calculating obesity [7].

1.2 Definition and types of dyslipidemia

Dyslipidemia is a medical condition characterized by abnormal levels of lipids in the blood. It is a major risk factor for cardiovascular disease, including heart attacks and strokes [8].

There are several types of dyslipidemia, including:

- High levels of low-density lipoprotein (LDL) cholesterol commonly referred to as "bad" cholesterol. LDL cholesterol can build up in the arteries, leading to plaque formation and narrowing of the blood vessels [9].

- Low levels of high-density lipoprotein (HDL) cholesterol commonly referred to as "good" cholesterol. HDL cholesterol helps remove excess cholesterol from the blood vessels and carries it to the liver for processing [10].

- High levels of triglycerides, which are another type of fat in the blood. High levels of triglycerides are often associated with low levels of HDL cholesterol and can increase the risk of cardiovascular disease [9].

- Combined dyslipidemia, which refers to having high levels of both LDL cholesterol and triglycerides and low levels of HDL cholesterol.

Dyslipidemia can be caused by several factors, including genetics, lifestyle factors such as diet and exercise, and certain medical conditions such as diabetes and hypothyroidism [8]. Treatment options for dyslipidemia include lifestyle modifications such as diet and exercise, as well as medications such as statins and fibrates [8].

1.3 Importance of leptin in energy balance and metabolism

Leptin, discovered in 1994, is a hormone that plays a key role in regulating energy balance and body weight [11]. It acts on the hypothalamus to suppress appetite and increase energy expenditure [12]. Leptin also influences lipid metabolism, including synthesis, storage, and transport [13]. By binding to receptors in the hypothalamus, leptin signals the brain about the body's fat stores and helps regulate food intake and energy expenditure [14, 15]. High leptin levels reduce food intake and increase energy expenditure, while low levels stimulate hunger and conserve energy [12]. Leptin also increases energy expenditure by activating the sympathetic nervous system [16]. Moreover, it enhances insulin sensitivity and glucose metabolism, reducing the risk of insulin resistance and diabetes [17]. Dysregulation of leptin signaling can contribute to obesity and metabolic disorders [14].

1.4 Significance of leptin resistance in obesity

Leptin resistance is a condition where cells become less responsive to the hormone leptin, resulting in an inability to regulate appetite and energy balance effectively [18]. In obesity, adipose tissue produce elevated levels of leptin, which should decrease appetite and increase energy expenditure to reduce body weight. However, many obese individuals experience inadequate brain response to increased leptin, leading to improper regulation of appetite and energy balance, known as leptin resistance [19].

Leptin resistance in obesity is believed to be caused by several factors, including chronic inflammation, insulin resistance, and changes in the hypothalamus and other brain regions that regulate appetite and energy balance. These factors can lead to a disruption in leptin signaling [20].

Leptin resistance can be a vicious cycle in obesity, as higher levels of fat stores lead to increased leptin production, which should reduce appetite and increase energy expenditure [21]. However, when leptin resistance occurs, the body fails to respond appropriately to the increased leptin levels, leading to continued overeating and reduced energy expenditure, contributing to further weight gain and worsening of the condition [22].

2. Leptin: physiology and mechanisms

2.1 Role of leptin in regulating appetite, energy expenditure, and metabolism

Leptin plays a crucial role in regulating appetite, energy expenditure, and metabolism.

Appetite regulation: When leptin levels rise, it signals to the brain that the body has enough energy stores and suppresses appetite. Conversely, when leptin levels are low, it signals hunger and increases appetite [23].

Energy expenditure: When leptin levels rise, it stimulates the production of energy-burning brown fat, which helps to burn calories and regulate body weight. Conversely, when leptin levels are low, the body conserves energy by reducing metabolic rate and storing fat [24].

Metabolism: Leptin also regulates metabolism by influencing the breakdown and storage of nutrients. It enhances the breakdown of stored fats in adipose tissue, promotes the conversion of glucose to energy, and reduces the production of glucose in the liver [24].

Leptin resistance, which occurs when the body becomes insensitive to the effects of leptin, can disrupt the balance of appetite, energy expenditure, and metabolism. This can lead to obesity, metabolic syndrome, and other health problems [23, 24].

2.2 Leptin signaling pathway and its effects on lipid metabolism

The leptin signaling pathway begins with the binding of leptin to its receptor, which is located on the surface of cells in the hypothalamus and other parts of the body. When leptin binds to its receptor, it activates a cascade of signaling molecules that transmit the signal into the cell, resulting in various physiological effects [25].

One of the main effects of leptin on lipid metabolism is the promotion of lipolysis, which is the breakdown of stored fat in adipose tissue. Leptin stimulates lipolysis by activating an enzyme called hormone-sensitive lipase (HSL), which breaks down triglycerides (stored fat) into free fatty acids and glycerol. The free fatty acids can then be used as a source of energy by other tissues in the body [26].

Leptin also affects lipid metabolism by regulating the expression of genes involved in lipid synthesis and storage. It inhibits the expression of genes involved in fatty acid synthesis, such as fatty acid synthase (FAS), and stimulates the expression of genes involved in fatty acid oxidation, such as carnitine palmitoyltransferase-1 (CPT-1). This results in a shift towards fat burning and away from fat storage [27].

Furthermore, leptin signaling affects the activity of several transcription factors, including peroxisome proliferator-activated receptor gamma (PPAR-gamma) and sterol regulatory element-binding protein-1c (SREBP-1c), which are key regulators of lipid metabolism. Leptin inhibits the activity of PPAR-gamma, which promotes fat storage, and stimulates the activity of SREBP-1c, which promotes fatty acid oxidation [28].

Leptin signaling pathway plays a crucial role in regulating lipid metabolism by promoting lipolysis, inhibiting fatty acid synthesis, and stimulating fatty acid oxidation. These effects help to maintain energy balance and prevent the development of metabolic disorders such as obesity and type 2 diabetes mellitus [29].

2.3 Leptin receptors and mechanisms of leptin action

Leptin, a hormone involved in metabolism and energy homeostasis, exerts its effects on various tissues throughout the body through specific mechanisms of action mediated by leptin receptors. The distribution of leptin receptors reflects the diverse effects of leptin on different tissues and highlights its crucial role in maintaining overall health and wellness [30, 31]. Leptin receptors are proteins that are expressed on the surface of various cells in the body and are responsible for binding and responding to the hormone leptin. There are six different isoforms of leptin receptors, which are generated by alternative splicing of the gene encoding the receptor. These isoforms differ in their length and structure, and some have different affinities for leptin [32].

In adipose tissue, leptin regulates the synthesis and release of adipokines, which are signaling molecules involved in metabolic processes such as inflammation and insulin sensitivity. Leptin also activates hormone-sensitive lipase (HSL), promoting lipolysis—the breakdown of stored fat into free fatty acids and glycerol. These fatty acids are then released into the bloodstream for energy production [11].

In the liver, leptin inhibits glucose synthesis and promotes the breakdown of stored glycogen. It also suppresses the synthesis of fatty acids and triglycerides, thus reducing the risk of fatty liver disease (hepatic steatosis) [33].

Leptin plays a role in skeletal muscle by promoting glucose uptake and metabolism. It activates AMP-activated protein kinase (AMPK), which increases glucose uptake and energy production in muscle cells. This process helps improve insulin sensitivity [34].

In the pancreas, leptin inhibits insulin secretion from pancreatic beta cells. By reducing insulin levels in the bloodstream, leptin helps prevent hyperinsulinemia and improves insulin sensitivity in peripheral tissues [35].

Leptin's action in the brain primarily occurs in the hypothalamus, where it regulates appetite, energy expenditure, and metabolism. Leptin suppresses the release of appetite-stimulating neuropeptide Y (NPY) and agouti-related peptide (AgRP), while stimulating the release of appetite-suppressing proopiomelanocortin (POMC) and cocaine-and-amphetamine-regulated transcript (CART). Additionally, leptin increases the activity of brown adipose tissue and promotes thermogenesis, thereby enhancing energy expenditure [36].

Overall, leptin's effects on specific tissues are mediated by leptin receptors, which are expressed in adipose tissue, liver, skeletal muscle, pancreas, and the hypothalamus of the brain. By understanding these tissue-specific mechanisms of action, we can better appreciate the role of leptin in regulating metabolism and maintaining energy balance.

3. Obesity: causes and risk factors

3.1 Causes for obesity

It is critical to pinpoint the causes of any medical illness to comprehend it properly. Obesity has a wide variety of underlying causes. These consist of the following [37]:

- *Gender:* Women are more prone to weight gain than men, potentially due to factors such as a slower metabolic rate and postmenopausal metabolic rate decline. Retaining weight gained during pregnancy is another contributing factor.
- *Heredity:* Obesity can run in families, suggesting a genetic contribution. Having an obese or overweight mother increases the risk of developing obesity. Genetic factors influence energy intake, expenditure, and susceptibility to obesity.
- *Genetics of obesity:* Carrying two copies of the FTO gene is associated with higher body weight and increased risk of obesity. The heritability of obesity varies, and polymorphisms in multiple genes can affect appetite and metabolism.
- *Unhealthy eating habits:* Regular consumption of a high-fat diet and junk food, large meals, and irregular eating schedules contribute to obesity. The relationship between fast food consumption and obesity is prominent.
- *Excessive calorie intake:* Overeating is prevalent worldwide, contributing to obesity. The proportion of obese adults has significantly increased over time.
- *Malnutrition:* Childhood malnutrition followed by the availability of additional dietary energy can promote fat accumulation. Certain foods and endocrine disruptors can alter lipid metabolism.
- *Endocrine disorders:* Certain endocrine disorders, such as growth hormone insufficiency, Cushing's disease, and hypothyroidism, can cause obesity.
- *Sedentary lifestyle:* Lack of physical activity and modern conveniences that reduce the need for physical exertion contribute to obesity. Reduced levels of physical activity in children and adults are concerning.
- *Psychological factors:* Emotional eating as a coping mechanism, binge eating due to depression, and stress-induced overeating contribute to obesity. Sleep deprivation is also a factor.
- *Psychiatric illness:* Eating disorders and specific mental conditions increase the risk of obesity.
- *Medications:* Some medications, such as insulin, antidepressants, steroids, and hormonal contraceptives, may lead to weight gain or body composition changes.

3.2 Risk factors for obesity

Some people develop a susceptibility to fat via no fault of their own. Several risk factors increase the chances of becoming obese. These consist of the following [1]:

- *Family history:* Heredity can play a role in obesity, but it is not solely due to genetics. Family eating habits and lifestyle choices can also contribute to the tendency for obesity to run in families. Children of two obese parents have a much higher risk of being obese.

- *Side effects of quitting smoking:* Some individuals may experience weight gain after quitting smoking, contributing to obesity. Former smokers may gain several pounds per week after quitting, with an average weight gain of 4 to 10 pounds in the first six months.

3.3 Pathophysiology of obesity

Obesity arises from an imbalance between energy intake and expenditure influenced by behavioral and physiological factors [38]. The surge in obesity rates in Western countries is primarily attributed to changing environmental conditions, including decreased exercise and possibly increased food intake [39]. Factors such as increased calorie intake, reduced energy expenditure, or a combination of both can contribute to obesity.

While sedentary behavior is believed to contribute to weight gain, more research is needed to establish this link conclusively [40]. Physical activity involvement tends to decline with age, with a higher percentage of women than men reporting insufficient exercise in each age group [41]. Other variables associated with being overweight include age, race, gender, and socioeconomic status, although the reasons for these associations are not fully understood [42]. The high heritability of body mass index suggests that genetics play a significant role in obesity [43]. The genetics and the environment contribute to 30 to 40% and 60 to 70% of the variance in BMI, respectively [44]. Genetic factors may interact with environmental conditions, such as high-fat diets and a sedentary lifestyle, to increase the risk of obesity [45].

Metabolic syndrome and fat intake are positively correlated, with high levels of cholesterol, saturated fat, and sugar commonly found in Western diets. Fatty acids and cholesterol have been linked to pro-inflammatory signaling cascades in cultured macrophages [46]. Genetic mutations in the pro-opiomelanocortin (POMC) gene can result in severe obesity by impairing the synthesis of Alpha-melanocyte-stimulating hormone (α-MSH), a neuropeptide that reduces hunger. Mutations in the proenzyme convertase 1 (PC-1) gene can also hinder the synthesis of α-MSH from its precursor peptide, POMC. The type 4 melanocortin receptor (MC4R) binds to α-MSH and plays a role in preventing overeating. Loss-of-function mutations in this receptor can contribute to extreme obesity in some individuals [47–49]. Leptin and its receptors are involved in regulating appetite and weight through the enhancement of α-MSH and POMC [50]. The environment plays a significant role in obesity, regardless of genetic predisposition, as evidenced by famine preventing obesity in susceptible individuals [50].

The lipostat regulatory system, which involves signals from energy stores compared to targets in the brain, determines food intake, activity levels, and metabolism. Some obese individuals may have excessively high lipostats, leading to excessive body weight. The concept of a body weight "set point" is supported by physiological mechanisms involving an adipostat receptor in the hypothalamus and a sensing system in adipose tissue that reflects fat storage [51]. The adipostat signal influences appetite and energy expenditure based on the body's fat reserves [52]. Leptin, produced by the Ob gene, and leptin receptors produced by the db gene are involved in this physiological regulation [11].

Hormones such as ghrelin, cholecystokinin, insulin, adiponectin, orexin, peptide YY (PYY 3–36) and other mediators play a role in hunger control, adipose tissue storage patterns, and the development of insulin resistance [53]. Adipokines, which are mediators produced by adipose tissue, are believed to influence various disorders associated with obesity [54]. Leptin, primarily released by adipose cells, acts on the brain and regulates long-term hunger. Ghrelin and leptin work in concert to impact short-term and long-term hunger signals [55–57].

Leptin and ghrelin specifically target the hypothalamus, a key brain region involved in hunger regulation. The melanocortin pathway in the hypothalamus, particularly the arcuate nucleus, plays a crucial role in controlling satiety and appetite. Neurons in the arcuate nucleus express agouti-related peptide/neuropeptide-Y (AgRP/NPY) and POMC cocaine-and-amphetamine-regulated-transcript (POMC/CART), with the former promoting feeding and the latter promoting satiety [58–60]. Leptin stimulates the POMC/CART neurons while inhibiting the AgRP/NPY neurons, contributing to the regulation of food intake. Leptin deficiency or resistance can lead to increased food intake and may contribute to certain forms of obesity [61].

3.4 Metabolic abnormalities associated with obesity, including dyslipidemia

Obesity is a complex metabolic disorder that is associated with several metabolic abnormalities, including dyslipidemia. Dyslipidemia is a condition characterized by abnormal levels of lipids (fats) in the blood, including high levels of low-density lipoprotein (LDL) cholesterol (commonly referred to as "bad" cholesterol), low levels of high-density lipoprotein (HDL) cholesterol (commonly referred to as "good" cholesterol), and high levels of triglycerides [62].

In obesity, the accumulation of excess fat in adipose tissue leads to dyslipidemia through several mechanisms. First, adipose tissue secretes pro-inflammatory cytokines and hormones, such as leptin and adiponectin, which can promote inflammation and insulin resistance. Insulin resistance can lead to increased production of very-low-density lipoprotein (VLDL) in the liver, which can contribute to increased levels of triglycerides in the blood [63].

Additionally, excess adipose tissue can lead to an increased production of LDL cholesterol particles and a decrease in HDL cholesterol levels. This can lead to the formation of atherosclerotic plaques in the blood vessels, increasing the risk of cardiovascular disease [64].

Obesity is also associated with changes in the gut microbiome, which can contribute to dyslipidemia. Changes in the gut microbiome can lead to an increase in the production of bile acids, which can contribute to increased cholesterol absorption in the gut [65].

Furthermore, obesity is often associated with a sedentary lifestyle and unhealthy dietary habits, such as a high intake of saturated and trans fats, which can contribute to dyslipidemia [64].

Dyslipidemia is a significant risk factor for cardiovascular disease, including heart attacks and strokes. Therefore, management of dyslipidemia is an important component of obesity treatment. Treatment options for dyslipidemia include lifestyle modifications such as diet and exercise, as well as medications such as statins and fibrates, which can help to lower LDL cholesterol levels and increase HDL cholesterol levels [64].

3.5 Role of adipose tissue in obesity-related metabolic dysregulation

Adipose tissue is a key component in the development of obesity-related metabolic dysfunctions. In obesity, the adipose tissue becomes dysfunctional, leading to chronic inflammation, insulin resistance, and dyslipidemia. One of the primary functions of adipose tissue is to store excess energy in the form of triglycerides. When the energy intake exceeds energy expenditure, the adipose tissue expands to accommodate the excess energy. In obesity, this expansion can lead to adipose tissue dysfunction, characterized by hypertrophy (increase in adipocyte size) and hyperplasia (increase in adipocyte number) [66].

Adipose tissue dysfunction can lead to the release of pro-inflammatory cytokines, such as TNF-alpha and IL-6, which can promote inflammation and insulin resistance. Insulin resistance occurs when cells become less responsive to insulin, leading to a decrease in glucose uptake and metabolism. This can lead to high blood sugar levels and eventually to the development of type 2 diabetes [67].

Furthermore, adipose tissue can release free fatty acids into the bloodstream, which can contribute to dyslipidemia. Free fatty acids can lead to an increase in triglycerides and LDL cholesterol levels, while also decreasing HDL cholesterol levels [68].

Additionally, adipose tissue produces several hormones, such as leptin and adiponectin, which can influence appetite and metabolism. Leptin, which is produced by adipocytes, regulates appetite and energy expenditure by signaling to the hypothalamus in the brain. However, in obesity, the body can become resistant to leptin, leading to a failure to regulate appetite and energy expenditure properly [52]. Adiponectin, on the other hand, plays a role in insulin sensitivity and glucose metabolism. In obesity, the production of adiponectin is often decreased, leading to a decrease in insulin sensitivity and an increase in blood sugar levels [69].

Overall, adipose tissue dysfunction plays a significant role in the development of obesity-related metabolic dysfunctions. Treatment strategies for obesity-related metabolic dysfunctions often involve lifestyle modifications, such as diet and exercise, as well as pharmacological interventions that target adipose tissue function and inflammation [70].

3.6 Overview of the concept of adipokines and their role in obesity

Adipokines are a group of bioactive molecules that are secreted by adipose tissue and play an important role in the regulation of energy metabolism, inflammation, and immune function. Adipokines can have both pro-inflammatory and anti-inflammatory effects, depending on the specific adipokine and the context in which it is secreted [71].

In obesity, adipose tissue becomes dysfunctional, leading to alterations in the secretion of adipokines. Dysregulated adipokine secretion can contribute to the development of obesity-related metabolic disorders, such as insulin resistance, dyslipidemia, and cardiovascular disease [72]. Leptin is one of the most well-known adipokines and is primarily secreted by adipocytes [18].

Adiponectin is another important adipokine that plays a role in insulin sensitivity and glucose metabolism. Adiponectin levels are typically decreased in obesity, contributing to insulin resistance and an increase in blood sugar levels [73]. Other adipokines, such as TNF-alpha, IL-6, and resistin, have been implicated in the development of inflammation and insulin resistance in obesity [74, 75]. TNF-alpha and IL-6 are pro-inflammatory cytokines that are secreted by adipose tissue and can contribute to the development of chronic inflammation, while resistin has been shown to impair insulin signaling [75]. On the other hand, adipokines such as omentin, visfatin, and adipolin have been shown to have anti-inflammatory effects and can improve insulin sensitivity [76].

Overall, the dysregulated secretion of adipokines in obesity plays a critical role in the development of metabolic dysfunctions. Understanding the mechanisms by which adipokines contribute to obesity-related disorders can help in the development of new therapeutic strategies for the prevention and treatment of obesity and its associated complications [66].

4. Dyslipidemia: pathophysiology and consequences

4.1 Pathophysiology of dyslipidemia, including the role of lipoproteins

Dyslipidemia is a common metabolic disorder characterized by an abnormal level of lipids (cholesterol and triglycerides) in the blood. It is a major risk factor for the development of cardiovascular disease, which remains the leading cause of morbidity and mortality worldwide. The pathophysiology of dyslipidemia is complex and involves an imbalance in the production and clearance of lipoproteins [9].

Lipoproteins are complexes of lipids and proteins that play a critical role in the transport of lipids in the bloodstream. They are classified into several types based on their density and size. The main types of lipoproteins include chylomicrons, very-low-density lipoproteins (VLDL), intermediate-density lipoproteins (IDL), low-density lipoproteins (LDL), and high-density lipoproteins (HDL) [77].

Chylomicrons are formed in the intestine and transport dietary triglycerides to the liver and peripheral tissues [78]. VLDL is synthesized in the liver and transports endogenous triglycerides to peripheral tissues [79]. IDL is a remnant of VLDL metabolism, and LDL is a remnant of IDL metabolism. LDL is often referred to as "bad" cholesterol because it can accumulate in the arterial wall and contribute to the development of atherosclerosis, a condition characterized by the buildup of plaque in the arteries. In contrast, HDL is often referred to as "good" cholesterol because it can remove excess cholesterol from peripheral tissues and transport it to the liver for elimination [80].

The pathophysiology of dyslipidemia involves an imbalance in the production and clearance of lipoproteins [81]. In insulin resistance and obesity, the liver produces an excess of VLDL, leading to elevated triglycerides in the blood. Elevated VLDL can also lead to an increase in LDL levels as VLDL is converted to LDL [82]. In addition to the overproduction of VLDL, dyslipidemia can also be caused by a decrease in LDL clearance. LDL particles can become modified, making them more prone to accumulate in the arterial wall and contribute to the development of atherosclerosis [83].

HDL levels are also affected in dyslipidemia. In insulin resistance and obesity, there is a decrease in HDL levels, which can contribute to the development of atherosclerosis [84]. HDL can become dysfunctional, losing its ability to remove excess cholesterol from peripheral tissues [85]. Overall, the dysregulation of lipoprotein metabolism in dyslipidemia plays a critical role in the development of atherosclerosis and cardiovascular disease [77].

Dyslipidemia is a complex metabolic disorder that is characterized by an abnormal level of lipids in the blood [86]. Lipoproteins, which are complexes of lipids and proteins, play a critical role in the transport of lipids in the bloodstream [78]. The pathophysiology of dyslipidemia involves an imbalance in the production and clearance of lipoproteins, leading to the accumulation of lipids in the arterial wall and the development of atherosclerosis [87]. Understanding the role of lipoproteins in dyslipidemia can help in the development of new therapeutic strategies for the prevention and treatment of cardiovascular disease [88].

4.2 Consequences of dyslipidemia on cardiovascular health, liver function, and other organs

Dyslipidemia is a significant risk factor for the development of cardiovascular disease, which remains the leading cause of morbidity and mortality worldwide. The consequences of dyslipidemia on cardiovascular health, liver function, and other organs are numerous and can be severe.

Consequences of dyslipidemia on cardiovascular health: Dyslipidemia can lead to the development of atherosclerosis, a condition characterized by the buildup of plaque in the arteries [77]. The accumulation of plaque can narrow the arteries, reducing blood flow to the heart and other organs. In severe cases, atherosclerosis can lead to the formation of blood clots that can block the arteries, leading to heart attacks, strokes, and other cardiovascular events [89]. Dyslipidemia is also associated with the development of hypertension, which is another significant risk factor for cardiovascular disease [90].

Consequences of dyslipidemia on liver function: The liver plays a critical role in the metabolism of lipids. In dyslipidemia, the liver can become overwhelmed by an excess of triglycerides and cholesterol, leading to the accumulation of fat in the liver (hepatic steatosis) [91]. Hepatic steatosis can progress to nonalcoholic steatohepatitis (NASH), a more severe form of liver disease that is associated with inflammation, fibrosis, and cirrhosis [92]. NASH can lead to liver failure and an increased risk of liver cancer [93].

Consequences of dyslipidemia on other organs: Dyslipidemia can also affect other organs, such as the pancreas, kidneys, and brain. In the pancreas, dyslipidemia can lead to the development of insulin resistance and type 2 diabetes mellitus [94]. Dyslipidemia is also associated with the development of chronic kidney disease, which can lead to kidney failure [95]. In the brain, dyslipidemia is associated with cognitive decline, dementia, and Alzheimer's disease [96].

4.3 Importance of managing dyslipidemia in the context of overall health

The management and prevention of dyslipidemia involve lifestyle modifications, such as a healthy diet, regular exercise, weight loss, and smoking cessation. Medications, such as statins, fibrates, niacin, and cholesterol absorption inhibitors, are also commonly used to lower lipid levels in the blood. The treatment of dyslipidemia can reduce the risk of cardiovascular disease and improve liver function, kidney function, and other organ health.

Dyslipidemia is a significant risk factor for the development of cardiovascular disease, liver disease, and other health complications. The consequences of dyslipidemia on cardiovascular health, liver function, and other organs can be severe and life-threatening. The management and prevention of dyslipidemia involve lifestyle modifications and medications. Early detection and treatment of dyslipidemia can reduce the risk of cardiovascular disease and improve overall health outcomes.

5. Leptin and dyslipidemia: mechanisms and interactions

5.1 Impact of leptin on lipid metabolism, including lipogenesis, lipolysis, and fatty acid oxidation

Leptin acts on various tissues in the body, including the liver, muscle, and adipose tissue, to influence lipid metabolism.

- *Impact of leptin on lipogenesis:* Leptin inhibits lipogenesis, the process of synthesizing new fatty acids from glucose. Leptin accomplishes this by suppressing the activity of enzymes that are involved in the synthesis of fatty acids, such as acetyl-CoA carboxylase and fatty acid synthase. Leptin also increases the activity of enzymes that are involved in the breakdown of fatty acids, such as hormone-sensitive lipase, thereby promoting lipolysis [97].

- *Impact of leptin on lipolysis:* Leptin promotes lipolysis, the process of breaking down triglycerides in adipose tissue into fatty acids and glycerol. Leptin accomplishes this by activating hormone-sensitive lipase, an enzyme that is involved in the breakdown of triglycerides in adipose tissue. The resulting increase in circulating fatty acids can be used as a source of energy by various tissues in the body, including muscle and liver [98].

- *Impact of leptin on fatty acid oxidation:* Leptin also promotes fatty acid oxidation, the process of using fatty acids as a source of energy. Leptin accomplishes this by increasing the expression of genes involved in fatty acid oxidation, such as peroxisome proliferator-activated receptor alpha (PPARα) and carnitine palmitoyltransferase I (CPT1). PPARα is a transcription factor that regulates the expression of genes involved in fatty acid oxidation, while CPT1 is an enzyme that transports fatty acids into the mitochondria, where they can be oxidized for energy production [99].

In summary, leptin plays a critical role in lipid metabolism by inhibiting lipogenesis, promoting lipolysis, and increasing fatty acid oxidation. Dysregulation of leptin signaling can contribute to the development of dyslipidemia, obesity, and related metabolic disorders. Understanding the impact of leptin on lipid metabolism may lead to the development of new therapies for the treatment of metabolic disorders.

5.2 Leptin's role in regulating hepatic lipid metabolism

Leptin acts on the liver to influence lipid metabolism, including lipogenesis, lipolysis, and fatty acid oxidation.

- *Role of leptin in hepatic lipogenesis:* Leptin inhibits hepatic lipogenesis, the process of synthesizing new fatty acids from glucose. Leptin accomplishes this by suppressing the activity of enzymes that are involved in the synthesis of fatty acids, such as acetyl-CoA carboxylase and fatty acid synthase [100]. In addition, leptin also reduces the expression of sterol regulatory element-binding protein 1c (SREBP-1c), a transcription factor that regulates the expression of genes involved in lipogenesis [18].

- *Role of leptin in hepatic lipolysis:* Leptin promotes hepatic lipolysis, the process of breaking down triglycerides stored in the liver into fatty acids and glycerol. Leptin accomplishes this by activating hormone-sensitive lipase, an enzyme that is involved in the breakdown of triglycerides in adipose tissue [11]. The resulting increase in circulating fatty acids can be used as a source of energy by various tissues in the body, including the liver.

- *Role of leptin in hepatic fatty acid oxidation:* Leptin also promotes hepatic fatty acid oxidation, the process of using fatty acids as a source of energy. Leptin accomplishes this by increasing the expression of genes involved in fatty acid oxidation, such as peroxisome proliferator-activated receptor alpha (PPARα) and carnitine palmitoyltransferase I (CPT1). PPARα is a transcription factor that regulates the expression of genes involved in fatty acid oxidation, while CPT1 is an enzyme that transports fatty acids into the mitochondria, where they can be oxidized for energy production [100].

Leptin resistance, a condition where the body is resistant to the effects of leptin, is associated with dysregulation of hepatic lipid metabolism. In individuals with leptin resistance, the liver may continue to produce and store fatty acids, leading to the development of hepatic steatosis, a condition characterized by the accumulation of fat in the liver [101]. Over time, hepatic steatosis can progress to nonalcoholic steatohepatitis (NASH), a more severe form of liver disease that can lead to liver fibrosis, cirrhosis, and hepatocellular carcinoma [102].

Leptin plays an essential role in regulating hepatic lipid metabolism by inhibiting lipogenesis, promoting lipolysis, and increasing fatty acid oxidation [103]. Dysregulation of leptin signaling can contribute to the development of hepatic steatosis and related liver disorders. Understanding the impact of leptin on hepatic lipid metabolism may lead to the development of new therapies for the treatment of liver diseases [104].

5.3 Influence of leptin resistance on lipid metabolism and dyslipidemia

Leptin resistance is a condition where the body is less sensitive to the effects of leptin. It is commonly seen in individuals with obesity and is thought to contribute to the development of dyslipidemia, a condition characterized by abnormal levels of lipids in the blood [105]. Leptin resistance can lead to dysregulation of lipid metabolism in several ways.

Firstly, leptin resistance can result in increased lipogenesis, the process of synthesizing new fatty acids from glucose. This is because leptin normally inhibits lipogenesis in the liver, but when leptin resistance occurs, this inhibitory effect is diminished [106]. As a result, the liver may continue to produce and store fatty acids, leading to the development of dyslipidemia.

Secondly, leptin resistance can contribute to decreased lipolysis, the process of breaking down stored triglycerides into fatty acids and glycerol. Leptin normally promotes lipolysis by activating hormone-sensitive lipase, an enzyme involved in the breakdown of stored triglycerides. However, when leptin resistance occurs, this activation is reduced, leading to decreased breakdown of stored triglycerides and a buildup of triglycerides in the blood [107].

Thirdly, leptin resistance can lead to decreased fatty acid oxidation, the process of using fatty acids as a source of energy. Leptin normally promotes fatty acid oxidation by increasing the expression of genes involved in fatty acid oxidation, such as peroxisome proliferator-activated receptor alpha (PPARα) and carnitine palmitoyl transferase I (CPT1). However, when leptin resistance occurs, this up regulation is reduced, leading to decreased fatty acid oxidation and a buildup of fatty acids in the blood [108]. All of these changes in lipid metabolism can contribute to the development of dyslipidemia, including increased levels of triglycerides, LDL cholesterol, and decreased levels of HDL cholesterol. Dyslipidemia is a major risk factor for cardiovascular disease, and therefore, leptin resistance can increase the risk of developing cardiovascular disease.

Leptin resistance is a condition that is commonly seen in individuals with obesity and can contribute to dyslipidemia by affecting lipid metabolism in several ways. Understanding the role of leptin resistance in dyslipidemia may lead to the development of new therapies for the treatment of dyslipidemia and its associated cardiovascular risks [75].

5.4 Interactions between leptin and other adipokines in the context of dyslipidemia

Leptin has been shown to interact with several other adipokines, including adiponectin, resistin, and visfatin [109]. Adiponectin is a protein hormone that is also secreted by adipose tissue and is known to have insulin-sensitizing and anti-inflammatory effects. Adiponectin has been shown to improve lipid metabolism by increasing fatty acid oxidation and decreasing lipogenesis. Additionally, adiponectin has been shown to inhibit the formation of foam cells, which are a key component of atherosclerotic plaques that contribute to the development of cardiovascular disease [110]. Leptin has been shown to have an inhibitory effect on adiponectin production, which may contribute to the dysregulation of lipid metabolism seen in individuals with leptin resistance [111].

Resistin is another adipokine that has been implicated in the development of dyslipidemia. Resistin is thought to contribute to the development of insulin resistance and dyslipidemia by decreasing insulin sensitivity and increasing lipolysis. Leptin has been shown to have a stimulatory effect on resistin production, which may further exacerbate the effects of resistin on lipid metabolism [112, 113].

Visfatin, also known as nicotinamidephosphoribosyltransferase (NAMPT), is another adipokine that has been shown to play a role in the regulation of lipid metabolism. Visfatin has been shown to increase lipolysis and decrease fatty acid oxidation, which can contribute to the development of dyslipidemia. Leptin has been shown to have a stimulatory effect on visfatin production, which may further contribute to the dysregulation of lipid metabolism seen in individuals with leptin resistance [114].

Interactions between leptin and other adipokines, such as adiponectin, resistin, and visfatin, are thought to play an important role in the development of dyslipidemia. Dysregulation of these interactions, particularly in the context of leptin resistance, may contribute to the development of dyslipidemia and its associated cardiovascular risks. Understanding the complex interplay between these adipokines may lead to the development of new therapies for the treatment of dyslipidemia and its associated complications.

6. Clinical implications and management

6.1 Clinical significance of leptin and dyslipidemia in obesity-related health outcomes

Leptin and dyslipidemia are two important factors that are associated with obesity-related health outcomes, and their clinical significance cannot be overstated. Leptin, as a hormone that is secreted by adipose tissue, plays a key role in regulating energy metabolism and appetite. In obesity, however, individuals often develop a resistance to leptin, which can lead to dysregulation of energy balance and metabolic dysfunction. This can lead to a range of health outcomes, including insulin resistance; type 2 diabetes mellitus, and cardiovascular disease [64, 75, 77, 90].

Dyslipidemia, on the other hand, refers to abnormalities in lipid metabolism, including elevated levels of cholesterol and triglycerides. Obesity is a major risk factor for dyslipidemia, as excess adipose tissue can lead to increased production of triglycerides and decreased clearance of cholesterol. Dyslipidemia can lead to the development of atherosclerosis and cardiovascular disease, which are major causes of morbidity and mortality in individuals with obesity [9, 10, 87, 88].

The clinical significance of leptin and dyslipidemia in obesity-related health outcomes can be seen in numerous studies [115–117]. For example, studies have shown that individuals with leptin resistance are at increased risk of developing type 2 diabetes, cardiovascular disease, and non-alcoholic fatty liver disease. Similarly, dyslipidemia has been linked to an increased risk of cardiovascular disease and other metabolic disorders in individuals with obesity [64, 70].

Treatment of leptin resistance and dyslipidemia is an important aspect of managing obesity-related health outcomes. Lifestyle modifications, such as dietary changes and increased physical activity, can improve both leptin resistance and dyslipidemia [118]. Medications, such as statins for dyslipidemia and leptin sensitizers for leptin resistance, may also be used in some cases [119, 120].

Leptin and dyslipidemia are both clinically significant factors in obesity-related health outcomes. Understanding their role in the development of metabolic dysfunction and cardiovascular disease is important in developing effective prevention and treatment strategies for individuals with obesity [121].

6.2 Diagnostic evaluation and assessment of dyslipidemia in the context of leptin and obesity

The diagnostic evaluation and assessment of dyslipidemia in the context of leptin and obesity typically involves a combination of clinical evaluation, laboratory testing, and imaging studies.

Clinical evaluation may include a detailed medical history and physical examination, which can help identify risk factors for dyslipidemia and cardiovascular disease. This may include a history of obesity, diabetes, hypertension, and family history of cardiovascular disease.

Laboratory testing is also an important component of the diagnostic evaluation for dyslipidemia. This typically includes a lipid profile, which measures levels of total cholesterol, LDL cholesterol, HDL cholesterol, and triglycerides in the blood. In individuals with obesity and/or leptin resistance, these levels may be elevated [122].

Imaging studies, such as computed tomography (CT) or magnetic resonance imaging (MRI), may also be used to assess the extent of fatty infiltration in the liver, which is a common complication of dyslipidemia in the context of obesity and leptin resistance [123].

In addition to these standard tests, assessment of leptin levels and leptin resistance may also be considered in individuals with obesity and dyslipidemia. This may involve measurement of circulating leptin levels, as well as assessment of leptin receptor expression and signaling in adipose tissue [105].

Overall, the diagnostic evaluation and assessment of dyslipidemia in the context of leptin and obesity should be tailored to the individual patient and may involve a multidisciplinary approach involving primary care physicians, endocrinologists, and cardiologists. The goal of this evaluation is to identify and address underlying metabolic dysfunctions in order to prevent or manage complications such as cardiovascular disease and non-alcoholic fatty liver disease.

6.3 Management approaches for dyslipidemia in obese individuals

The management of dyslipidemia in obese individuals typically involves a combination of lifestyle modifications, pharmacotherapy, and bariatric surgery, depending on the severity of the dyslipidemia and the presence of other risk factors for cardiovascular disease.

Lifestyle modifications: Lifestyle modifications are the first line of treatment for dyslipidemia in obese individuals. This may include dietary changes such as reducing intake of saturated and trans fats, increasing fiber intake, and reducing overall caloric intake. Regular physical activity is also important, with a goal of at least 150 minutes of moderate-intensity exercise per week. Weight loss through caloric restriction and increased physical activity can also improve dyslipidemia in obese individuals [119].

Pharmacotherapy: In some cases, lifestyle modifications may not be enough to manage dyslipidemia in obese individuals. In these cases, pharmacotherapy may be necessary. The most commonly used medications for dyslipidemia are statins, which work by inhibiting the production of cholesterol in the liver. Other medications such as ezetimibe, niacin, and fibrates may also be used alone or in combination with statins [124].

Bariatric surgery: Bariatric surgery, such as gastric bypass or sleeve gastrectomy, may also be considered in obese individuals with severe dyslipidemia who have not responded to lifestyle modifications and/or pharmacotherapy. Bariatric surgery can improve dyslipidemia by promoting weight loss and improving insulin sensitivity. However, it is important to note that bariatric surgery is a major surgical procedure and is not without risks [125].

It is important to note that the management of dyslipidemia in obese individuals should be individualized and tailored to the specific needs and medical history of the patient. Close monitoring of lipid levels, as well as any potential side effects of medications, is also important in ensuring effective management of dyslipidemia in this population.

7. Future directions and emerging therapies targeting leptin and dyslipidemia in obesity

Leptin and dyslipidemia are both complex metabolic conditions that are closely related to obesity. While current treatments, including lifestyle modifications, pharmacotherapy, and bariatric surgery, can be effective in managing dyslipidemia in obese individuals, emerging therapies targeting leptin and dyslipidemia hold promise for improving outcomes [126]. One potential approach involves targeting leptin resistance directly. Leptin sensitizers, such as the drug metreleptin, have been shown to improve insulin sensitivity and lipid metabolism in patients with leptin deficiency [127]. More research is needed to determine whether these drugs could be effective in treating leptin resistance in obese individuals.

Another approach involves targeting specific adipokines that play a role in dyslipidemia. For example, the drug adipotide, which targets the adipokine adiponectin, has been shown to reduce body weight and improve insulin sensitivity in animal models. Clinical trials are currently underway to determine whether adipotide could be effective in treating obesity-related conditions in humans [128].

Other emerging therapies include gene therapy, stem cell therapy, and microbiome-based therapies. Gene therapy approaches involving the introduction of genes regulating lipid metabolism into adipose tissue are being explored. These strategies aim to address dyslipidemia in obesity by directly targeting adipose tissue. Further research is needed to evaluate the efficacy and safety of gene therapy in managing dyslipidemia [129]. Stem cell therapy may involve using stem cells to regenerate healthy adipose tissue or to promote lipid metabolism. This approach aims to address dyslipidemia in obesity by leveraging the regenerative capabilities of stem cells [130]. Microbiome-based therapies, which involve manipulating the gut microbiota, have shown promise in promoting healthy lipid metabolism. These approaches seek to modulate dyslipidemia by targeting the gut microbiome. Further research is needed to determine the efficacy and mechanisms of microbiome-based therapies in managing dyslipidemia [131].

Overall, the development of new therapies targeting leptin and dyslipidemia in obesity is an active area of research. While these therapies are still in the early stages of development, they hold promise for improving outcomes for individuals with obesity-related metabolic conditions.

8. Conclusion

Dyslipidemia is a condition characterized by abnormal levels of lipids, such as cholesterol and triglycerides, in the blood. It is a major risk factor for cardiovascular diseases, including atherosclerosis, heart attack, and stroke. Leptin, a hormone primarily produced by adipose tissue, has been found to play a significant role in dyslipidemia.

One of the key mechanisms through which leptin affects lipid metabolism is by inhibiting the synthesis of fatty acids in adipose tissue. Leptin reduces the activity of an enzyme called fatty acid synthase, which is responsible for converting excess glucose into fatty acids for storage in adipose tissue. By inhibiting this enzyme, leptin helps to reduce the accumulation of fatty acids in adipose tissue and prevent the development of obesity.

Leptin also plays a role in regulating lipid transport in the blood. It has been shown to increase the clearance of triglycerides from the blood by enhancing the uptake and metabolism of triglyceride-rich lipoproteins by the liver. Leptin also promotes the breakdown of triglycerides stored in adipose tissue, releasing fatty acids into the blood to be used as an energy source by other tissues.

Furthermore, leptin has been found to have anti-inflammatory effects, which can have a positive impact on dyslipidemia. Leptin reduces the production of pro-inflammatory cytokines in adipose tissue and liver, which are known to contribute to the development of insulin resistance and atherosclerosis.

Leptin also stimulates the production of anti-inflammatory cytokines, which can help to reduce inflammation and improve lipid metabolism. However, in conditions of obesity; leptin resistance can develop, leading to decreased sensitivity to the effects of leptin. This can result in an imbalance in lipid metabolism and contribute to dyslipidemia.

Acknowledgements

The authors would like to acknowledge Haveri Institute of Medical Sciences, Haveri and St. George's University School of Medicine, St. George's, Grenada for their support.

Conflict of interest

The authors declare no conflict of interest.

Notes/thanks/other declarations

Nil.

Author details

Harish Rangareddy[1*], Priyanka Venkatapathappa[2], Kesava Mandalaneni[3], Ashakiran Srinivasaiah[1] and Katherine Bourne-Yearwood[4]

1 Department of Biochemistry, Haveri Institute of Medical Sciences, Haveri, Karnataka, India

2 Department of University Health Services, St. George's University, St. George's, Grenada

3 Department of Neuroscience and Behavioral Sciences, St. George's University School of Medicine, St. George's, Grenada

4 University Health Sciences, St. George's University, St. Georges', Grenada

*Address all correspondence to: harishreddy1349@gmail.com

References

[1] Boutari C, Mantzoros CS. A 2022 update on the epidemiology of obesity and a call to action: as its twin COVID-19 pandemic appears to be receding, the obesity and dysmetabolism pandemic continues to rage on. Metabolism. 2022;**133**:155217. DOI: 10.1016/j.metabol.2022.155217 Epub 2022 May 15

[2] Loos RJ, Bouchard C. Obesity--is it a genetic disorder? Journal of Internal Medicine. 2003;**254**(5):401-425. DOI: 10.1046/j.1365-2796.2003.01242.x

[3] World Health Organization. Body Mass Index - BMI. Geneva: World Health Organization; 2021

[4] Després JP. Body fat distribution and risk of cardiovascular disease: An update. Circulation. 2012;**126**(10):1301-1313. DOI: 10.1161/CIRCULATIONAHA.111.067264

[5] Bhaskaran K, Dos-Santos-Silva I, Leon DA, Douglas IJ, Smeeth L. Association of BMI with overall and cause-specific mortality: A population-based cohort study of 3·6 million adults in the UK. The Lancet Diabetes and Endocrinology. 2018;**6**(12):944-953. DOI: 10.1016/S2213-8587(18)30288-2 Epub 2018 Oct 30

[6] Lynn W, Agrawal S. Introduction to obesity. In: Obesity, Bariatric and Metabolic Surgery: A Comprehensive Guide. Cham: Springer International Publishing; 2021. pp. 1-12

[7] Bray GA, Kim KK, Wilding JPH. Obesity: A Chronic Relapsing Progressive Disease Process. A Position Statement of the World Obesity Federation. London: World Obesity Federation; 2017

[8] Ganda OP. Dyslipidemia: Pathophysiology, evaluation, and management. In: Feingold KR, Anawalt B, Boyce A, et al., editors. Endotext. South Dartmouth (MA): MDText.com, Inc.; 2000

[9] Nordestgaard BG, Varbo A. Triglycerides and cardiovascular disease. Lancet. 2014;**384**(9943):626-635. DOI: 10.1016/S0140-6736(14)61177-6

[10] Rader DJ, Hovingh GK. HDL and cardiovascular disease. Lancet. 2014;**384**(9943):618-625. DOI: 10.1016/S0140-6736(14)61217-4

[11] Zhang Y, Proenca R, Maffei M, Barone M, Leopold L, Friedman JM. Positional cloning of the mouse obese gene and its human homologue. Nature. 1994;**372**(6505):425-432. DOI: 10.1038/372425a0 Erratum in: Nature 1995;374(6521):479

[12] Farooqi IS, Bullmore E, Keogh J, Gillard J, O'Rahilly S, Fletcher PC. Leptin regulates striatal regions and human eating behavior. Science. 2007;**317**(5843):1355. DOI: 10.1126/science.1144599 Epub 2007 Aug 9

[13] Münzberg H, Jobst EE, Bates SH, Jones J, Villanueva E, Leshan R, et al. Appropriate inhibition of orexigenic hypothalamic arcuate nucleus neurons independently of leptin receptor/STAT3 signaling. The Journal of Neuroscience. 2007;**27**(1):69-74. DOI: 10.1523/JNEUROSCI.3168-06.2007

[14] Myers MG Jr, Heymsfield SB, Haft C, Kahn BB, Laughlin M, Leibel RL, et al. Challenges and opportunities of defining clinical leptin resistance. Cell Metabolism. 2012;**15**(2):150-156. DOI: 10.1016/j.cmet.2012.01.002

[15] El-Haschimi K, Pierroz DD, Hileman SM, Bjørbaek C, Flier JS. Two

defects contribute to hypothalamic leptin resistance in mice with diet-induced obesity. The Journal of Clinical Investigation. 2000;**105**(12):1827-1832. DOI: 10.1172/JCI9842

[16] Münzberg H, Flier JS, Bjørbaek C. Region-specific leptin resistance within the hypothalamus of diet-induced obese mice. Endocrinology. 2004;**145**(11):4880-4889. DOI: 10.1210/en.2004-0726 Epub 2004 Jul 22

[17] Morton GJ, Cummings DE, Baskin DG, Barsh GS, Schwartz MW. Central nervous system control of food intake and body weight. Nature. 2006;**443**(7109):289-295. DOI: 10.1038/nature05026

[18] Ahima RS, Flier JS. Leptin. Annual Review of Physiology. 2000;**62**:413-437. DOI: 10.1146/annurev.physiol.62.1.413

[19] Myers MG Jr, Leibel RL, Seeley RJ, Schwartz MW. Obesity and leptin resistance: Distinguishing cause from effect. Trends in Endocrinology and Metabolism. 2010;**21**(11):643-651. DOI: 10.1016/j.tem.2010.08.002 Epub 2010 Sep 16

[20] Bjørbaek C, Kahn BB. Leptin signaling in the central nervous system and the periphery. Recent Progress in Hormone Research. 2004;**59**:305-331. DOI: 10.1210/rp.59.1.305

[21] Briggs DI, Lockie SH, Benzler J, Wu Q, Stark R, Reichenbach A, et al. Evidence that diet-induced hyperleptinemia, but not hypothalamic gliosis, causes ghrelin resistance in NPY/AgRP neurons of male mice. Endocrinology. 2014;**155**(7):2411-2422. DOI: 10.1210/en.2013-1861 Epub 2014 Apr 17

[22] Morton GJ, Schwartz MW. Leptin and the central nervous system control of glucose metabolism. Physiological Reviews. 2011;**91**(2):389-411. DOI: 10.1152/physrev.00007.2010

[23] Ahima RS. Revisiting leptin's role in obesity and weight loss. The Journal of Clinical Investigation. 2008;**118**(7):2380-2383. DOI: 10.1172/JCI36284

[24] Morrison CD. Leptin signaling in brain: A link between nutrition and cognition? Biochimica et Biophysica Acta. 2009;**1792**(5):401-408. DOI: 10.1016/j.bbadis.2008.12.004 Epub 2008 Dec 24

[25] Davis JF, Choi DL, Schurdak JD, Fitzgerald MF, Clegg DJ, Lipton JW, et al. Leptin regulates energy balance and motivation through action at distinct neural circuits. Biological Psychiatry. 2011;**69**(7):668-674. DOI: 10.1016/j.biopsych.2010.08.028 Epub 2010 Oct 29

[26] Martínez-Sánchez N. There and Back again: Leptin actions in White adipose tissue. International Journal of Molecular Sciences. 2020;**21**(17):6039. DOI: 10.3390/ijms21176039

[27] Gastaldelli A, Gaggini M, DeFronzo RA. Role of adipose tissue insulin resistance in the natural history of type 2 diabetes: Results from the San Antonio metabolism study. Diabetes. 2017;**66**(4):815-822. DOI: 10.2337/db16-1167 Epub 2017 Jan 4

[28] Faggioni R, Feingold KR, Grunfeld C. Leptin regulation of the immune response and the immunodeficiency of malnutrition. The FASEB Journal. 2001;**15**(14):2565-2571. DOI: 10.1096/fj.01-0431rev

[29] Minokoshi Y, Kim YB, Peroni OD, Fryer LG, Müller C, Carling D, et al. Leptin stimulates fatty-acid oxidation by activating AMP-activated protein

kinase. Nature. 2002;**415**(6869):339-343. DOI: 10.1038/415339a

[30] Paz-Filho G, Mastronardi C, Franco CB, Wang KB, Wong ML, Licinio J. Leptin: Molecular mechanisms, systemic pro-inflammatory effects, and clinical implications. Arquivos Brasileiros de Endocrinologia e Metabologia. 2012;**56**(9):597-607. DOI: 10.1590/s0004-27302012000900001

[31] Margetic S, Gazzola C, Pegg GG, Hill RA. Leptin: A review of its peripheral actions and interactions. International Journal of Obesity and Related Metabolic Disorders. 2002;**26**(11):1407-1433. DOI: 10.1038/sj.ijo.0802142

[32] Myers MG Jr, Olson DP. Central nervous system control of metabolism. Nature. 2012;**491**(7424):357-363. DOI: 10.1038/nature11705

[33] Steinberg GR, Parolin ML, Heigenhauser GJ, Dyck DJ. Leptin increases FA oxidation in lean but not obese human skeletal muscle: Evidence of peripheral leptin resistance. American Journal of Physiology. Endocrinology and Metabolism. 2002;**283**(1):E187-E192. DOI: 10.1152/ajpendo.00542.2001

[34] Shi H, Strader AD, Woods SC, Seeley RJ. The effect of fat removal on glucose tolerance is depot specific in male and female mice. American Journal of Physiology. Endocrinology and Metabolism. 2007;**293**(4):E1012-E1020. DOI: 10.1152/ajpendo.00649.2006 Epub 2007 Jul 24

[35] Ahima RS, Antwi DA. Brain regulation of appetite and satiety. Endocrinology and Metabolism Clinics of North America. 2008;**37**(4):811-823. DOI: 10.1016/j.ecl.2008.08.005

[36] Münzberg H, Morrison CD. Structure, production and signaling of leptin. Metabolism. 2015;**64**(1):13-23. DOI: 10.1016/j.metabol.2014.09.010 Epub 2014 Sep 28

[37] Casazza K, Fontaine KR, Astrup A, Birch LL, Brown AW, Bohan Brown MM, et al. Myths, presumptions, and facts about obesity. The New England Journal of Medicine. 2013;**368**(5):446-454. DOI: 10.1056/NEJMsa1208051

[38] Bray GA, Frühbeck G, Ryan DH, Wilding JP. Management of obesity. Lancet. 2016;**387**(10031):1947-1956. DOI: 10.1016/S0140-6736(16)00271-3 Epub 2016 Feb 10

[39] Hill JO, Wyatt HR, Reed GW, Peters JC. Obesity and the environment: Where do we go from here? Science. 2003;**299**(5608):853-855. DOI: 10.1126/science.1079857

[40] King GA, Fitzhugh EC, Bassett DR Jr, McLaughlin JE, Strath SJ, Swartz AM, et al. Relationship of leisure-time physical activity and occupational activity to the prevalence of obesity. International Journal of Obesity and Related Metabolic Disorders. 2001;**25**(5):606-612. DOI: 10.1038/sj.ijo.0801583

[41] Surgeon General's report on physical activity and health. From the Centers for Disease Control and Prevention. Journal of the American Medical Association. 1996;**276**(7):522

[42] Ogden CL, Carroll MD, Kit BK, Flegal KM. Prevalence of obesity and trends in body mass index among US children and adolescents, 1999-2010. Journal of the American Medical Association. 2012;**307**(5):483-490. DOI: 10.1001/jama.2012.40 Epub 2012 Jan 17

[43] Bouchard C, Tremblay A, Després JP, Nadeau A, Lupien PJ, Thériault G, et al.

The response to long-term overfeeding in identical twins. The New England Journal of Medicine. 1990;**322**(21):1477-1482. DOI: 10.1056/NEJM199005243222101

[44] Maes HH, Neale MC, Eaves LJ. Genetic and environmental factors in relative body weight and human adiposity. Behavior Genetics. 1997;**27**(4):325-351. DOI: 10.1023/a:1025635913927

[45] Frayling TM. Genome-wide association studies provide new insights into type 2 diabetes aetiology. Nature Reviews. Genetics. 2007;**8**(9):657-662. DOI: 10.1038/nrg2178

[46] Després JP. Health consequences of visceral obesity. Annals of Medicine. 2001;**33**(8):534-541. DOI: 10.3109/07853890108995963

[47] Krude H, Biebermann H, Luck W, Horn R, Brabant G, Grüters A. Severe early-onset obesity, adrenal insufficiency and red hair pigmentation caused by POMC mutations in humans. Nature Genetics. 1998;**19**(2):155-157. DOI: 10.1038/509

[48] Cone RD. Anatomy and regulation of the central melanocortin system. Nature Neuroscience. 2005;**8**(5):571-578. DOI: 10.1038/nn1455

[49] Vaisse C, Clement K, Durand E, Hercberg S, Guy-Grand B, Froguel P. Melanocortin-4 receptor mutations are a frequent and heterogeneous cause of morbid obesity. The Journal of Clinical Investigation. 2000;**106**(2):253-262. DOI: 10.1172/JCI9238

[50] Farooqi IS, Keogh JM, Yeo GS, Lank EJ, Cheetham T, O'Rahilly S. Clinical spectrum of obesity and mutations in the melanocortin 4 receptor gene. The New England Journal of Medicine. 2003;**348**(12):1085-1095. DOI: 10.1056/NEJMoa022050

[51] van Son J, Koekkoek LL, La Fleur SE, Serlie MJ, Nieuwdorp M. The role of the gut microbiota in the gut-brain Axis in obesity: Mechanisms and future implications. International Journal of Molecular Sciences. 2021;**22**(6):2993. DOI: 10.3390/ijms22062993

[52] Friedman JM, Halaas JL. Leptin and the regulation of body weight in mammals. Nature. 1998;**395**(6704):763-770. DOI: 10.1038/27376

[53] Druce M, Bloom SR. The regulation of appetite. Archives of Disease in Childhood. 2006;**91**(2):183-187. DOI: 10.1136/adc.2005.073759

[54] Bray GA, Tartaglia LA. Medicinal strategies in the treatment of obesity. Nature. 2000;**404**(6778):672-677. DOI: 10.1038/35007544

[55] Chen H, Charlat O, Tartaglia LA, Woolf EA, Weng X, Ellis SJ, et al. Evidence that the diabetes gene encodes the leptin receptor: Identification of a mutation in the leptin receptor gene in db/db mice. Cell. 1996;**84**(3):491-495. DOI: 10.1016/s0092-8674(00)81294-5

[56] Clément K, Vaisse C, Lahlou N, Cabrol S, Pelloux V, Cassuto D, et al. A mutation in the human leptin receptor gene causes obesity and pituitary dysfunction. Nature. 1998;**392**(6674):398-401. DOI: 10.1038/32911

[57] Cui H, López M, Rahmouni K. The cellular and molecular bases of leptin and ghrelin resistance in obesity. Nature Reviews. Endocrinology. 2017;**13**(6):338-351. DOI: 10.1038/nrendo.2016.222 Epub 2017 Feb 24

[58] Farooqi IS, O'Rahilly S. Leptin: A pivotal regulator of human

energy homeostasis. The American Journal of Clinical Nutrition. 2009;**89**(3):980S-984S. DOI: 10.3945/ajcn.2008.26788C Epub 2009 Feb 11

[59] Cummings DE, Foster-Schubert KE, Overduin J. Ghrelin and energy balance: Focus on current controversies. Current Drug Targets. 2005;**6**(2):153-169. DOI: 10.2174/1389450053174569

[60] Elmquist JK, Elias CF, Saper CB. From lesions to leptin: Hypothalamic control of food intake and body weight. Neuron. 1999;**22**(2):221-232. DOI: 10.1016/s0896-6273(00)81084-3

[61] Cowley MA, Smart JL, Rubinstein M, Cerdán MG, Diano S, Horvath TL, et al. Leptin activates anorexigenic POMC neurons through a neural network in the arcuate nucleus. Nature. 2001;**411**(6836):480-484. DOI: 10.1038/35078085

[62] Grundy SM. Obesity, metabolic syndrome, and cardiovascular disease. The Journal of Clinical Endocrinology and Metabolism. 2004;**89**(6):2595-2600. DOI: 10.1210/jc.2004-0372

[63] Licata G, Argano C, Di Chiara T, Parrinello G, Scaglione R. Obesity: A main factor of metabolic syndrome? Panminerva Medica. 2006;**48**(2):77-85

[64] Eckel RH, Alberti KG, Grundy SM, Zimmet PZ. The metabolic syndrome. Lancet. 2010;**375**(9710):181-183. DOI: 10.1016/S0140-6736(09)61794-3

[65] Turnbaugh PJ, Ley RE, Mahowald MA, Magrini V, Mardis ER, Gordon JI. An obesity-associated gut microbiome with increased capacity for energy harvest. Nature. 2006;**444**(7122):1027-1031. DOI: 10.1038/nature05414

[66] Trayhurn P, Wood IS. Signalling role of adipose tissue: Adipokines and inflammation in obesity. Biochemical Society Transactions. 2005;**33**(Pt 5):1078-1081. DOI: 10.1042/BST0331078

[67] Sun K, Kusminski CM, Scherer PE. Adipose tissue remodeling and obesity. The Journal of Clinical Investigation. 2011;**121**(6):2094-2101. DOI: 10.1172/JCI45887 Epub 2011 Jun 1

[68] Shoelson SE, Herrero L, Naaz A. Obesity, inflammation, and insulin resistance. Gastroenterology. 2007;**132**(6):2169-2180. DOI: 10.1053/j.gastro.2007.03.059

[69] Kadowaki T, Yamauchi T. Adiponectin and adiponectin receptors. Endocrine Reviews. 2005;**26**(3):439-451. DOI: 10.1210/er.2005-0005

[70] Després JP, Lemieux I. Abdominal obesity and metabolic syndrome. Nature. 2006;**444**(7121):881-887. DOI: 10.1038/nature05488

[71] Ouchi N, Parker JL, Lugus JJ, Walsh K. Adipokines in inflammation and metabolic disease. Nature Reviews. Immunology. 2011;**11**(2):85-97. DOI: 10.1038/nri2921 Epub 2011 Jan 21

[72] Blüher M. Adipose tissue dysfunction in obesity. Experimental and Clinical Endocrinology & Diabetes. 2009;**117**(6):241-250. DOI: 10.1055/s-0029-1192044 Epub 2009 Apr 8

[73] Yamauchi T, Kadowaki T. Adiponectin receptor as a key player in healthy longevity and obesity-related diseases. Cell Metabolism. 2013;**17**(2):185-196. DOI: 10.1016/j.cmet.2013.01.001 Epub 2013 Jan 24

[74] Hotamisligil GS, Shargill NS, Spiegelman BM. Adipose expression of tumor necrosis factor-alpha: Direct role in obesity-linked insulin resistance.

Science. 1993;**259**(5091):87-91. DOI: 10.1126/science.7678183

[75] Steppan CM, Bailey ST, Bhat S, Brown EJ, Banerjee RR, Wright CM, et al. The hormone resistin links obesity to diabetes. Nature. 2001;**409**(6818):307-312. DOI: 10.1038/35053000

[76] Kishida K, Kim KK, Funahashi T, Matsuzawa Y, Kang HC, Shimomura I. Relationships between circulating adiponectin levels and fat distribution in obese subjects. Journal of Atherosclerosis and Thrombosis. 2011;**18**(7):592-595. DOI: 10.5551/jat.7625 Epub 2011 Mar 3

[77] Ference BA, Ginsberg HN, Graham I, Ray KK, Packard CJ, Bruckert E, et al. Low-density lipoproteins cause atherosclerotic cardiovascular disease. 1. Evidence from genetic, epidemiologic, and clinical studies. A consensus statement from the European atherosclerosis society consensus panel. European Heart Journal. 2017;**38**(32):2459-2472. DOI: 10.1093/eurheartj/ehx144

[78] Hussain MM, Rava P, Walsh M, Rana M, Iqbal J. Multiple functions of microsomal triglyceride transfer protein. Nutrition & Metabolism (London). 2012;**9**:14. DOI: 10.1186/1743-7075-9-14

[79] Wiegman A, Hutten BA, de Groot E, Rodenburg J, Bakker HD, Büller HR, et al. Efficacy and safety of statin therapy in children with familial hypercholesterolemia: A randomized controlled trial. Journal of the American Medical Association. 2004;**292**(3):331-337. DOI: 10.1001/jama.292.3.331

[80] Brown MS, Goldstein JL. A receptor-mediated pathway for cholesterol homeostasis. Science. 1986;**232**(4746):34-47. DOI: 10.1126/science.3513311

[81] Emerging Risk Factors Collaboration, Di Angelantonio E, Sarwar N, Perry P, Kaptoge S, Ray KK, et al. Major lipids, apolipoproteins, and risk of vascular disease. Journal of the American Medical Association. 2009;**302**(18):1993-2000. DOI: 10.1001/jama.2009.1619

[82] Rashid S, Barrett PH, Uffelman KD, Watanabe T, Adeli K, Lewis GF. Lipolytically modified triglyceride-enriched HDLs are rapidly cleared from the circulation. Arteriosclerosis, Thrombosis, and Vascular Biology. 2002;**22**(3):483-487. DOI: 10.1161/hq0302.105374

[83] Libby P, Ridker PM, Hansson GK, Leducq Transatlantic Network on Atherothrombosis. Inflammation in atherosclerosis: From pathophysiology to practice. Journal of the American College of Cardiology. 2009;**54**(23):2129-2138. DOI: 10.1016/j.jacc.2009.09.009

[84] Kontush A, Chapman MJ. Antiatherogenic small, dense HDL--guardian angel of the arterial wall? Nature Clinical Practice. Cardiovascular Medicine. 2006;**3**(3):144-153. DOI: 10.1038/ncpcardio0500

[85] Rye KA, Barter PJ. Formation and metabolism of prebeta-migrating, lipid-poor apolipoprotein A-I. Arteriosclerosis, Thrombosis, and Vascular Biology. 2004;**24**(3):421-428. DOI: 10.1161/01.ATV.0000104029.74961.f5 Epub 2003 Oct 30

[86] Virani SS, Alonso A, Aparicio HJ, Benjamin EJ, Bittencourt MS, Callaway CW, et al. Heart disease and stroke Statistics-2021 update: A report from the American Heart Association. Circulation. 2021;**143**(8):e254-e743. DOI: 10.1161/CIR.0000000000000950 Epub 2021 Jan 27

[87] Stein EA. Low-density lipoprotein cholesterol reduction and prevention

of cardiovascular disease. Mayo Clinic Proceedings. 2009;**84**(4):307-309. DOI: 10.1016/S0025-6196(11)60537-5

[88] Mora S, Wenger NK, Cook NR, Liu J, Howard BV, Limacher MC, et al. Evaluation of the pooled cohort risk equations for cardiovascular risk prediction in a multiethnic cohort from the Women's Health Initiative. JAMA Internal Medicine. 2018;**178**(9):1231-1240. DOI: 10.1001/jamainternmed.2018.2875

[89] Hansson GK. Inflammation, atherosclerosis, and coronary artery disease. The New England Journal of Medicine. 2005;**352**(16):1685-1695. DOI: 10.1056/NEJMra043430

[90] Toth PP. Subclinical atherosclerosis: What it is, what it means and what we can do about it. International Journal of Clinical Practice. 2008;**62**(8):1246-1254. DOI: 10.1111/j.1742-1241.2008.01804.x Epub 2008 Jun 28

[91] Browning JD, Horton JD. Molecular mediators of hepatic steatosis and liver injury. The Journal of Clinical Investigation. 2004;**114**(2):147-152. DOI: 10.1172/JCI22422

[92] Chalasani N, Younossi Z, Lavine JE, Charlton M, Cusi K, Rinella M, et al. The diagnosis and management of nonalcoholic fatty liver disease: Practice guidance from the American Association for the Study of Liver Diseases. Hepatology. 2018;**67**(1):328-357. DOI: 10.1002/hep.29367 Epub 2017 Sep 29

[93] Caldwell SH, Crespo DM. The spectrum expanded: Cryptogenic cirrhosis and the natural history of non-alcoholic fatty liver disease. Journal of Hepatology. 2004;**40**(4):578-584. DOI: 10.1016/j.jhep.2004.02.013

[94] Donath MY, Shoelson SE. Type 2 diabetes as an inflammatory disease. Nature Reviews. Immunology. 2011;**11**(2):98-107. DOI: 10.1038/nri2925 Epub 2011 Jan 14

[95] Liang X, Ye M, Tao M, Zheng D, Cai R, Zhu Y, et al. The association between dyslipidemia and the incidence of chronic kidney disease in the general Zhejiang population: A retrospective study. BMC Nephrology. 2020;**21**(1):252. DOI: 10.1186/s12882-020-01907-5

[96] Cheng YW, Chiu MJ, Chen YF, Cheng TW, Lai YM, Chen TF. The contribution of vascular risk factors in neurodegenerative disorders: From mild cognitive impairment to Alzheimer's disease. Alzheimer's Research & Therapy. 2020;**12**(1):91. DOI: 10.1186/s13195-020-00658-7

[97] Yang Q, Graham TE, Mody N, Preitner F, Peroni OD, Zabolotny JM, et al. Serum retinol binding protein 4 contributes to insulin resistance in obesity and type 2 diabetes. Nature. 2005;**436**(7049):356-362. DOI: 10.1038/nature03711

[98] Harris RB. Direct and indirect effects of leptin on adipocyte metabolism. Biochimica et Biophysica Acta. 2014;**1842**(3):414-423. DOI: 10.1016/j.bbadis.2013.05.009 Epub 2013 May 17

[99] Wang MY, Lee Y, Unger RH. Novel form of lipolysis induced by leptin. The Journal of Biological Chemistry. 1999;**274**(25):17541-17544. DOI: 10.1074/jbc.274.25.17541

[100] Shimomura I, Hammer RE, Ikemoto S, Brown MS, Goldstein JL. Leptin reverses insulin resistance and diabetes mellitus in mice with congenital lipodystrophy. Nature. 1999;**401**(6748):73-76. DOI: 10.1038/43448

[101] Tilg H, Moschen AR. Evolution of inflammation in nonalcoholic fatty liver disease: The multiple parallel hits hypothesis. Hepatology. 2010;**52**(5):1836-1846. DOI: 10.1002/hep.24001

[102] Younossi ZM, Stepanova M, Afendy M, Fang Y, Younossi Y, Mir H, et al. Changes in the prevalence of the most common causes of chronic liver diseases in the United States from 1988 to 2008. Clinical Gastroenterology and Hepatology. 2011;**9**(6):524-530.e1; quiz e60. DOI: 10.1016/j.cgh.2011.03.020 Epub 2011 Mar 25

[103] Buettner C, Muse ED, Cheng A, Chen L, Scherer T, Pocai A, et al. Leptin controls adipose tissue lipogenesis via central, STAT3-independent mechanisms. Nature Medicine. 2008;**14**(6):667-675. DOI: 10.1038/nm1775 Epub 2008 Jun 1

[104] Saxena NK, Titus MA, Ding X, Floyd J, Srinivasan S, Sitaraman SV, et al. Leptin as a novel profibrogenic cytokine in hepatic stellate cells: Mitogenesis and inhibition of apoptosis mediated by extracellular regulated kinase (Erk) and Akt phosphorylation. The FASEB Journal. 2004;**18**(13):1612-1614. DOI: 10.1096/fj.04-1847fje Epub 2004 Aug 19

[105] Considine RV, Sinha MK, Heiman ML, Kriauciunas A, Stephens TW, Nyce MR, et al. Serum immunoreactive-leptin concentrations in normal-weight and obese humans. The New England Journal of Medicine. 1996;**334**(5):292-295. DOI: 10.1056/NEJM199602013340503

[106] Isaia GC, D'Amelio P, Di Bella S, Tamone C. Is leptin the link between fat and bone mass? Journal of Endocrinological Investigation. 2005;**28**(10 Suppl):61-65

[107] Maffei M, Fei H, Lee GH, Dani C, Leroy P, Zhang Y, et al. Increased expression in adipocytes of Ob RNA in mice with lesions of the hypothalamus and with mutations at the db locus. Proceedings of the National Academy of Sciences of the United States of America. 1995;**92**(15):6957-6960. DOI: 10.1073/pnas.92.15.6957

[108] Caro JF, Kolaczynski JW, Nyce MR, Ohannesian JP, Opentanova I, Goldman WH, et al. Decreased cerebrospinal-fluid/serum leptin ratio in obesity: A possible mechanism for leptin resistance. Lancet. 1996;**348**(9021):159-161. DOI: 10.1016/s0140-6736(96)03173-x

[109] Trayhurn P. Endocrine and signalling role of adipose tissue: New perspectives on fat. Acta Physiologica Scandinavica. 2005;**184**(4):285-293. DOI: 10.1111/j.1365-201X.2005.01468.x

[110] Yamauchi T, Kamon J, Ito Y, Tsuchida A, Yokomizo T, Kita S, et al. Cloning of adiponectin receptors that mediate antidiabetic metabolic effects. Nature. 2003;**423**(6941):762-769. DOI: 10.1038/nature01705 Erratum in: Nature. 2004 Oct 28;431(7012):1123

[111] Weyer C, Funahashi T, Tanaka S, Hotta K, Matsuzawa Y, Pratley RE, et al. Hypoadiponectinemia in obesity and type 2 diabetes: Close association with insulin resistance and hyperinsulinemia. The Journal of Clinical Endocrinology and Metabolism. 2001;**86**(5):1930-1935. DOI: 10.1210/jcem.86.5.7463

[112] Steppan CM, Lazar MA. Resistin and obesity-associated insulin resistance. Trends in Endocrinology and Metabolism. 2002;**13**(1):18-23. DOI: 10.1016/s1043-2760(01)00522-7

[113] Rajala MW, Obici S, Scherer PE, Rossetti L. Adipose-derived resistin and gut-derived resistin-like molecule-beta selectively impair insulin action

on glucose production. The Journal of Clinical Investigation. 2003;**111**(2):225-230. DOI: 10.1172/JCI16521

[114] Dahl TB, Holm S, Aukrust P, Halvorsen B. Visfatin/NAMPT: A multifaceted molecule with diverse roles in physiology and pathophysiology. Annual Review of Nutrition. 2012;**32**:229-243. DOI: 10.1146/annurev-nutr-071811-150746 Epub 2012 Mar 29

[115] Ahima RS. Adipose tissue as an endocrine organ. Obesity (Silver Spring). 2006;**14**(Suppl. 5):242S-249S. DOI: 10.1038/oby.2006.317

[116] Blüher S, Mantzoros CS. Leptin in humans: Lessons from translational research. The American Journal of Clinical Nutrition. 2009;**89**(3):991S-997S. DOI: 10.3945/ajcn.2008.26788E Epub 2009 Jan 28

[117] Turer AT, Scherer PE. Adiponectin: Mechanistic insights and clinical implications. Diabetologia. 2012;**55**(9):2319-2326. DOI: 10.1007/s00125-012-2598-x Epub 2012 Jun 12

[118] Look AHEAD Research Group, Wing RR. Long-term effects of a lifestyle intervention on weight and cardiovascular risk factors in individuals with type 2 diabetes mellitus: Four-year results of the look AHEAD trial. Archives of Internal Medicine. 2010;**170**(17):1566-1575. DOI: 10.1001/archinternmed.2010.334

[119] Authors/Task Force Members, Catapano AL, Graham I, De Backer G, Wiklund O, Chapman MJ, et al. ESC/EAS guidelines for the Management of Dyslipidaemias: The task force for the Management of Dyslipidaemias of the European Society of Cardiology (ESC) and European atherosclerosis society (EAS) developed with the special contribution of the European Assocciation for Cardiovascular Prevention & Rehabilitation (EACPR). Atherosclerosis. 2016;**2016**(253):281-344. DOI: 10.1016/j.atherosclerosis.2016.08.018 Epub 2016 Sep 1

[120] Obradovic M, Sudar-Milovanovic E, Soskic S, Essack M, Arya S, Stewart AJ, et al. Leptin and obesity: Role and clinical implication. Front Endocrinol (Lausanne). 2021;**12**:585887. DOI: 10.3389/fendo.2021.585887

[121] Bastien M, Poirier P, Lemieux I, Després JP. Overview of epidemiology and contribution of obesity to cardiovascular disease. Progress in Cardiovascular Diseases. 2014;**56**(4):369-381. DOI: 10.1016/j.pcad.2013.10.016 Epub 2013 Oct 24

[122] Grundy SM, Cleeman JI, Daniels SR, Donato KA, Eckel RH, Franklin BA, et al. Diagnosis and management of the metabolic syndrome: An American Heart Association/National Heart, Lung, and Blood Institute scientific statement. Circulation. 2005;**112**(17):2735-2752. DOI: 10.1161/CIRCULATIONAHA.105.169404 Epub 2005 Sep 12. Erratum in: Circulation. 2005;112(17):e297

[123] Ekstedt M, Franzén LE, Mathiesen UL, Thorelius L, Holmqvist M, Bodemar G, et al. Long-term follow-up of patients with NAFLD and elevated liver enzymes. Hepatology. 2006;**44**(4):865-873. DOI: 10.1002/hep.21327

[124] Stone NJ, Robinson JG, Lichtenstein AH, Bairey Merz CN, Blum CB, Eckel RH, et al. ACC/AHA guideline on the treatment of blood cholesterol to reduce atherosclerotic cardiovascular risk in adults: A report of the American College of Cardiology/American Heart Association task force

on practice guidelines. Journal of the American College of Cardiology. 2013, 2014;**63**(25 Pt B):2889-2934. DOI: 10.1016/j.jacc.2013.11.002 Epub 2013 Nov 12. Erratum in: J Am Coll Cardiol. 2014;63(25 Pt B):3024-3025. Erratum in: J Am Coll Cardiol. 2015 Dec 22;66(24):2812

[125] Puzziferri N, Roshek TB 3rd, Mayo HG, Gallagher R, Belle SH, Livingston EH. Long-term follow-up after bariatric surgery: A systematic review. Journal of the American Medical Association. 2014;**312**(9):934-942. DOI:10.1001/jama.2014.10706

[126] Licinio J, Caglayan S, Ozata M, Yildiz BO, de Miranda PB, O'Kirwan F, et al. Phenotypic effects of leptin replacement on morbid obesity, diabetes mellitus, hypogonadism, and behavior in leptin-deficient adults. Proceedings of the National Academy of Sciences of the United States of America. 2004;**101**(13):4531-4536. DOI: 10.1073/pnas.0308767101 Epub 2004 Mar 9

[127] Brown RJ, Valencia A, Startzell M, Cochran E, Walter PJ, Garraffo HM, et al. Metreleptin-mediated improvements in insulin sensitivity are independent of food intake in humans with lipodystrophy. The Journal of Clinical Investigation. 2018;**128**(8):3504-3516. DOI: 10.1172/JCI95476 Epub 2018 Jul 16

[128] Al-Ghadban S, Bunnell BA. Adipose tissue-derived stem cells: Immunomodulatory effects and therapeutic potential. Physiology (Bethesda, Md.). 2020;**35**(2):125-133. DOI: 10.1152/physiol.00021.2019

[129] Smith SJ, Cases S, Jensen DR, Chen HC, Sande E, Tow B, et al. Obesity resistance and multiple mechanisms of triglyceride synthesis in mice lacking Dgat. Nature Genetics. 2000;**25**(1):87-90. DOI: 10.1038/75651

[130] Tam CS, Lecoultre V, Ravussin E. Brown adipose tissue: Mechanisms and potential therapeutic targets. Circulation. 2012;**125**(22):2782-2791. DOI: 10.1161/CIRCULATIONAHA.111.042929

[131] Pedersen HK, Gudmundsdottir V, Nielsen HB, Hyotylainen T, Nielsen T, Jensen BA, et al. Human gut microbes impact host serum metabolome and insulin sensitivity. Nature. 2016;**535**(7612):376-381. DOI: 10.1038/nature18646 Epub 2016 Jul 13

Chapter 4

The Effect of a Walking Training Program at the LIPOXmax Point on the Body Mass Index in Male Type II Diabetes in the 40–60 Age Group

Rafik Hadj Aissa, Aissa Bait and Mohamed Guettaf

Abstract

The study aims to identify the effect of a training program by walking to the point LIPOXmax on the BMI of male diabetics (type II); we relied on the experimental approach because of its adequacy with the study, while the study sample was composed of 12 people with type II, which were randomly selected from the study population. We used the pre- and post-measurement of the training program using an impedancemetry device to measure the body mass index, as well as calculating the LIPOXmax walking rhythm, which varies from one patient to another. Finally, the results of the study showed that walking to the point LIPOXmax positively affects the reduction in the body mass index in men with type II diabetes in age group 40–60 years old.

Keywords: training program, type II diabetes, LIPOXmax, walking sport, body mass index (BMI)

1. Introduction

The health level of the people is one of the most important indicators of the advancement and progress of countries. That is why many developed countries seek to provide various services to their members, including providing health care, for all ages, in an effort to make money and effort. They are sure that this will bring benefits to them in the short- and long-term. Where human health can be likened to a regression line that tends from top to bottom, when the whole life of the individual is activity, vitality and happiness; this means that health is located at a point above the line, but when health is at a point on the line and in the direction down, most of his daily activities may stop [1]. The underlying relationship between the behavior of individuals and health, led to major transformations in the last three decades of the twentieth century, in the understanding and development of health, and the possibility of its impact on the individual level. Therefore, health education is one of the most important areas of modern public health, and is considered an essential part of any public health program [2]. For this reason, studying and understanding behavioral practices belonging to health, in its various directions, is the first step towards the process of planning for them and finding ways to develop them, which ultimately reflects on healthy growth, and this is in line with what the World Health Organization (WHO) advocates. In the same context, this organization was confirmed by the report of Dr. Alaa Alwan: Efforts must be focused on the prevention and treatment of classes of global killers, including diabetes mellitus [3]. The prevalence of diabetes for the last 30 years has been considered a significant increase among the world's population to the extent that it has become a real danger [4]. The global prevalence of diabetes in adults (aged 20–79 years) will be 6.4%, affecting 285 million adults in 2010, and will rise to 7.7% and 439 million adults by 2030. Between 2010 and 2030, there will be a 69% increase in the number of adults with diabetes in developing countries and 20% in developed countries [5]. According to some predictive studies, which conclude: a 2010 study, which concluded that the prevalence of diabetes in adults globally (ages 20–79 years) is 6.4%, and may affect 285 million adults in 2010, and could increase to 7.7%, or 439 million adults by 2030. Between 2010 and 2030, there will be a 69% increase in the number of adults with diabetes in developing countries and 20% in developed countries [5]. According to another study, the prevalence of diabetes for all age groups worldwide was estimated at 2.8% in 2000 and 4.4% in 2030. It is also expected that the total number of people with diabetes will increase from 171 million in 2000 to 366 million in 2030 [4]. On September 16, 2022, the World Health Organization announced on its official website: The number of people with diabetes increased from 108 million in 1980 to 422 million in 2014. In high-income countries [6], this meant that the current stats far exceeded what was expected. According to the World Diabetes Federation, which states in 2021 that 537 million adults (20–79 years) suffer from diabetes, 1 in 10 people, and this number is expected to reach 643 million by 2030. According to the same source, about 2 million people suffer from diabetes. Diabetes in Algeria, according to the 2021 report of the International Diabetes Federation (FID) and published in the framework of World Diabetes Day [7]. That diabetes mellitus is a health problem that affects the life of an insulin-dependent person. While there is general agreement on the value of physical activity in the prevention and management of many diseases, it is considered among the therapeutic tools in daily medical practice. It is also difficult to convince long-term inactive patients to engage in regular physical activity [8]. Walking is one of the practices that have emerged to achieve a better lifestyle, as it reflects the safety of the heart and lungs, and walking is among the sports recommended by the World Health Organization [7]. Up to the age of 65, the activity practiced can be of a moderately intense aerobic nature (aerobic exercise, cycling, and running), but practiced regularly. For example, it is possible to program 150–300 min per week if the effort is of moderate intensity [7]. Classification of physical activities: light intensity between 25 and 30% VO2 max, moderate intensity between 40 and 50% VO2 max [9]. There are many methods of treatment to reduce the level of sugar in the blood, such as reducing some materials rich in fats and some drugs that work to reduce the level of glucose in the blood, as well as walking briskly, which are considered among the means of treatment, and are easy to implement and do not have side effects such as medicines. Medium-intensity physical activity helps reduce body fat, and with very simple steps, the body can burn approximately 60 calories per 1.2 km compared to burning calories in the normal state of the body, but if the speed increases by 2.8 km in 30 minutes, the body will burn 200 calories [10]. The walking rhythm of LIPOXmax is also used in training when weight loss is necessary for overweight people, to adjust exercise intensity and load in diabetic patients [11]. The LIPOXmaxcorresponds to the intensity of exercise for which the oxidation of lipids is maximal. This metabolic index is determined by calorimetry during a progressive stress test. LIPOXmax can be used as a training target in various pathologies, including obesity and diabetes [12]. A [13] in 2002, under the title: Determining the intensity of exercise that leads to maximum fat oxidation, the aim of this study was to develop a test protocol to determine the intensity of exercise in which the rate of fat oxidation is at. Eighteen moderately trained cyclists performed a graded-fatigue exercise test, with 5-minute phases in 35-watt increments, four to six continuous prolonged (CE) tests performed at constant work rates, corresponding to GE test work rates were applied on separate days. Seven other subjects were given three different GE tests to exhaustion. Lipid oxidation was measured using indirect calorimeters, (indirect calorimetry). It is concluded that a protocol with phases (3 min) per phase and 35 W increments of work rate can be used to determine (maximal) fat oxidation. Fat oxidation rates are high over a wide range of intensity (LIPOXmax). However, with high-intensity (maximum) exercise, fat oxidation rates are significantly reduced [13]. An exercise intensity of 40%, VO2 max is sometimes used to target LIPOXmax training [12]. The body mass index, (IMC) "Indice de Masse Corporelle" formerly called the (Quenelle) index, is a measure of indicating nutritional status in adults, defined as a person's weight (kg) divided by the square of a person's height in meters (kg/m^2)), and the mathematical equation is as follows:

$$\text{BMI} = \text{weight}(\text{kg}) / \text{height}(\text{m})^2 \tag{1}$$

BMI is based on the effect of excess body fat and is highly associated with obesity. BMI was developed as an indicator of disease risk. With an increase in BMI, some of the common conditions related to overweight and obesity include cardiovascular disease, high blood pressure, and diabetes, etc. [14].

Many studies have dealt with the subject of studying walking and its relationship to health in patients with diabetes and obesity on different samples, including:

A study Mohammed Zerf, in 2019, under the title: Effects of walking training performed using continuous and interval methods on weight loss as effective strategies among postpartum women, to estimate the effect of walking intensity (interval training vs. traditional cardio) on postpartum weight loss. Materials and methods: A total of 39 postpartum women participated in this study. Moderate obese BMI and high-risk waist circumference, first births at the same school and social status. Subjects participated in this study to lose excess weight within three months of giving birth. Results: Our results indicate that interval training with brisk walking is a powerful tool for developing effective weight loss management strategies. Conclusions: That postpartum woman, who use walking to amplify their weight loss, use the following exercise program: at least three sets of 400 m (wf $\approx$ SR) × 5 per day, nine 400 m (wf $\approx$ SR) × 5 sets per week, and 36 sets of 400 m (wf $\approx$ SR) × 5 per month [15].

A study Achten. J, Gleeson. M, Jeukendrup. A.E in 2002, under the title: Determining the intensity of exercise that leads to maximum fat oxidation. The aim of this study was to develop a test protocol to determine the intensity of exercise in which the rate of fat oxidation is at methods: Eighteen moderately trained cyclists performed a graded-fatigue exercise test, with 5-minute phases in 35-watt increments, four to six continuous prolonged (CE) tests performed at constant work rates, and corresponding to GE test work rates were applied on separate days. Seven other subjects were given three different GE tests to exhaustion. Lipid oxidation was measured using indirect calorimeters, (indirect calorimetry). Conclusions: It is concluded that a protocol with phases (3 min) per phase and 35 W increments of work rate can be used to determine (maximal) fat oxidation. Fat oxidation rates are elevated over a wide range of intensity (LIPOXmax). However, with high-intensity (maximum) exercise, fat oxidation rates are significantly reduced [13].

A study Monique Mendelson, Michel Guinot, Anne Favre-Juvin, Bernard Wuyam, and Patrice Flore, in 2014, under the title: Methodological aspects of LIPOXmax measurement: Application conditions for people with metabolic pathologies. Lipoxmax corresponds to the exercise intensity for which lipid oxidation is maximal. This metabolic index is determined by calorimetry during a progressive stress test. Lipoxmax can be used as a training target in various pathologies, including obesity and diabetes. The objective of this review of question is to state the methodological aspects of the measurement of the LIPOXmax by paying a particular attention to the validity of the gaseous exchanges, the particularities of the protocol of determination, and the factors of variability and reliability. Secondly, the interest and feasibility of adapted physical activities targeting LIPOXmax in people with metabolic disorders will be explored [12].

2. Theoretical framework

2.1 The problem statement

Despite the importance of walking for diabetes, we noticed patients resorting to medicines directly, and through the results of previous studies, we need field studies for different societies, to highlight the benefit of walking, to be a scientific addition that can benefit this group of patients, as well as access to Experimental facts regarding this type of adapted program. Therefore, the problem of the study is:

Can walking exercise at (LIPOXmax) point contribute to the effect on body mass index (BMI) in patients with type II diabetes (40–60 years)?

2.2 The significance of the study

The importance of the study was also represented in the fact that individuals do not feel danger to their health except when they pass the danger stage of body weight, but this is not very important if we know that the major problem is the increase in the percentage of fat in our bodies, which appears on the morphology of our bodies after large accumulations, and because of its symptoms Negative effects on the health of the individual, the causes of which are due to laziness, lethargy, lack of physical activity, and malnutrition.

2.3 Study objectives

Among the objectives of the study is to identify the physical activity represented by the activity of walking, which has a physical and psychological health impact, as this activity is suitable for different ages and for both sexes, and it can be performed at any time and in all available spaces, and at a lower cost so that anyone can reap the benefits and fruits of sports. Health through a simple and easy program that ensures moving many parts of his body on a regular basis and for a specific period. Providing a precisely tuned program for practicing physical activities for this group, and adjusting the correct rhythm for each patient, when practicing walking, and this is according to the characteristics of each individual.

3. Methodology

3.1 Exploratory study

The association which monitors diabetics at the level of the wilaya of Laghouat was contacted, in order to tap into the database of patients registered at the level of the municipality of Laghouat. When the study population has been identified (all patients with type II diabetes) for the purpose of determining the study sample, which comprises 10% of the total study population.

Subsequently, we contacted the patients, in order to persuade them to practice physical activity, in particular walking, without specifying or explaining the main objective of this study (in order to exclude psychological effects on the sample of the study).

Since the nature of the subject determines the choice of the method used and based on the subject of our study, we must follow the experimental method.

3.2 Research group and sample

The population studied consisted of all diabetic patients (type II) residing in the municipality of Laghouat. Their number was determined by the social association of the wilaya of Laghouat of diabetics, and they are about 120 patients with type II diabetes, whose age varies between (40–60 years).

The sample members consist of people with diabetes mellitus (type II), as we selected the sample in a simple random way represented by 10% of the population, which included 12 men, whose ages ranged between (40–60 years old).

At the end of the study, the results of the subjects who underwent pre- and post-tests were taken into account, and they did not miss the sessions of the adapted program. Where the researchers applied the program to (20) patients from the study community, but at the end of the program (08) individuals were excluded due to their interruption of the program several times, that is. more than (03) absences whose results are not taken into account in the study. As for the control sample, its presence brings a positive methodological complement, which testifies to the results of the experimental sample, but it was not retained for the following reasons:

The psychological pressures experienced by diabetics and the difficulty in convincing them to participate in this type of study. The comparison of the results of the pretest and the posttest of the experimental sample can give a clear picture of the results of the pilot program and be sufficient for approval.

3.3 Fields of study

This experiment extended for a period of 3 months from 01/01/2019 to 31/03/2019, starting from conducting the pretests up to the posttest.

This study was carried out at the level of the municipal stadium of Laghouat (Abdelkader Ben Hamid).

3.4 Data collection tools

Used devices:

- Tanita Impedancemeter BC-545 N.

- It measures body mass index and other measurements.
- Heart rate monitor (cardiofréquencemètre KHALANJI).
- Calculating the walking pace at (LIPOXmax), an exercise intensity of 40%, VO2 max was used to target LIPOXmax training [12].

This experiment extended for a period of 03 months from 01/01/2019 to 31/03/2019, starting from conducting the pretests up to the posttest.

The measures proposed in the study were presented to a group of specialists (from sports training, biomedical aspect of sport, and doctor), and they agreed on the relevance of the measures and the method of their application, as well as how to implement the program proposed for this category in order to achieve the objectives set without exposing the health of the members of the sample to loads that could affect their health.

Test programming: We conducted the pre-measurements one day before applying the program, where the sample members were collected, and how to make the measurements and the application of the program were explained, and the same measurements were applied to all sample members (12 patients), and the sample members were subjected to the same post-measurements one day after the end of the program, that is. after 03 months.

3.5 Program time and content

See **Table 1.**

	Progressive intermediate cycle.						
Weeks	**Tuesday**	**Wednesday**	**Thursday**	**Friday**	**Saturday**	**Sunday**	**Monday**
01/01/2019	Mesures anthropométriques						
S1	47 mn			47 mn			47 mn
S2	50 mn			50 mn			50 mn
S3	43 mn		43 mn		43 mn		43 mn
S4	48 mn		48 mn		48 mn		48 mn
S5	53 mn		53 mn		53 mn		53 mn
S6	58 mn		58 mn		58 mn		58 mn
S7	58 mn	58 mn		58 mn		58 mn	58 mn
S8	54 mn	54 mn		54 mn	54 mn		54 mn
S9	58 mn	58 mn		58 mn		58 mn	58 mn
S10	58 mn	58 mn		58 mn		58 mn	58 mn
S11	58 mn	58 mn		58 mn		58 mn	58 mn
S12	52 mn	52 mn		52 mn	52 mn	52 mn	52 mn
24/03/2019	Mesures anthropométriques						

Source: Authors, 2022.

Table 1.
The time for the suggested walking sessions in terms of weeks.

Program time: The proposed walking training program was applied for a period of (12 weeks), meaning a period of 03 months, from Tuesday 01/01/2019 to Sunday 24/03/2019, between (03 training units per week) and (06 training units per week). This is according to the requirements of the program, as well as the characteristics of the patients. Between 150 and 300 minutes per week of moderate intensity were programmed.

Note: Follow the muscle stretches for (10 minutes) after each walking session.

Statistical tools: In order to verify the hypotheses, the study conducted a statistical study using the SPSS program, through which the obtained data were processed, as it included: the arithmetic mean, the standard deviation, and the T-test.

4. The applied aspect

See **Table 2.**

4.1 Analysis and discussion

From the results in **Table 2**, we note that the arithmetic mean of the pre-measurement scores, the body mass index measurement in the body is (24.31) with a standard deviation of (1.94). The arithmetic mean value of the post-measurement for the same group is (27) with a standard deviation of (1.82) and the value of the difference between the arithmetic mean between the pre- and post-measurements was (2.69), and this indicates that there are differences between the two measurements, and this is justified by the value of the T-test, whose value amounted to (–22.5) at the significance level of (0.00), which is less than the value (0.05), and this result proves that there are statistically significant differences between the scores of the pre-measurement and the scores of the post-measurement of the BMI of the experimental group.

Walking exercise at (LIPOXmax) had a positive effect on the body mass index of patients with type II diabetes (40–60 years), where the results of the statistical

Body mass index measurement.		
	Experimental sample	
	Pretest	**Posttest**
Number	12	12
Arithmetic mean	24.31	27.00
Standard deviation	1.94	1.82
	Difference between the averages	2.69
	T-value	–22.5
	Significance level	0.00
	Degrees of freedom	22
	Statistical significance	Significant

Source: Authors, 2022.

Table 2.
Significance of differences in measuring body mass index between the pretest and the posttest for the experimental group.

analysis showed that there were statistically significant differences between the pre-and post-measurement of the body mass index. This indicates that the decrease in BMI could be due to the content of the walking activity program applied to this sample, which is mainly based on walking exercises at LIPOXmax. This explains the possibility of the LIPOXmax walking program affecting the percentage of fat in the body. And from it, it is the one that affected the body mass index, and this is consistent with the study [10], which shows that regular walking leads to the prevention of obesity in patients with obesity. Diabetes reduces relative weight and improves body mass index levels in the age group 30–50 years. It also agrees with the study of [13], whose results concluded that the rates of fat oxidation rise over a wide range of LIPOXmax intensity, by using a special protocol to control this intensity.

It also agrees with the study [16], which says that physical activity in patients with diabetes (type II) with a diet leads to an improvement in cardiorespiratory fitness and a decrease in body mass index. A study [17] showed that walking in diabetic patients has a positive effect on the health of patients through a decrease in biological blood values, and it also improves flexibility, endurance, heart work, and weight reduction, in addition to a decrease in body mass index.

And from it, we can say that we have answered the study's question, the practice of walking at the "LIPOXmax" point has a positive effect on the body mass index of patients with type II diabetes (40–60 years).

Through the results of the study, we concluded that brisk walking is the optimal pace to reach the appropriate intensity at the LIPOXmax point for a group (40–60 years old) of diabetic patients who do not practice physical activity. It is the lack of regular physical activity that explains the observed elevation of the heart rate at the slightest movement or physical activity, especially if it is associated with weight gain, which elevates the heart rate at rest compared to people practicing physical activity on a regular basis. Walking at LIPOXmax represents the values of maximum heart rate and resting heart rate, and from this the study sample, based on the movements resulting from brisk walking, which stimulate the body to reach LIPOXmax and thus burning the greatest percentage of body fat. Unlike regular exercisers, who may need a little more effort to reach the fat oxidation peak, that is. the LIPOXmax point.

5. Conclusions

From what we have found, we can say that the application of an adapted program accompanying this group of patients, which focuses on walking at the "LIPOXmax" point, has proven effective in helping diabetics in reducing body fat percentage and thus controlling excess body weight. The study showed that it is enough to practice walking alone without the need for fast running, or high-intensity physical activities, or anaerobic activities, to control the complications resulting from excess body fat in patients with type II diabetes.

From it, it can be said that the first goal that we seek is to promote a healthy lifestyle to combat the effects of type II diabetes and to benefit from the dissemination of sports culture with scientific standards, especially for those with diabetes who have excess weight.

Author details

Rafik Hadj Aissa*, Aissa Bait and Mohamed Guettaf
University Amar Telidji, Laghouat, Algeria

*Address all correspondence to: r.hadjaissa@lagh-univ.dz

References

[1] Salama YZM. Health attitudes and their relationship to health behavior among Benha University Students [master's thesis]. Benha University-Faculty of Physical Education-Department of Sports Health Sciences; 2012

[2] Billat V. Révolution Marathon. France: Amazon France; 2018

[3] World Health Organization. WHO Takes Stock of Non-communicable Diseases in All Countries. Geneva: Media Centre; 2011. Available from: https://www.who.int/mediacentre/news/releases/2011/NCDs_profiles_20110914/en/

[4] Wild S, Roglic G, Green A, Sicree R, King H. Global prevalence of diabetes, estimates for the year 2000 and projections for 2030. Diabetes Care. 2004;**27**(5):1051

[5] Shaw JE, Sicree RA, Zimmet ZP. Global estimates of the prevalence of diabetes for 2010 and 2030. Diabetes Research and Clinical Practice. 2010;**87**(1):4-14

[6] World Health Organization. How Much of Physical Activity is Recommended?, Newsroom, Geneva. 2022. Available from: https://www.who.int/news-room/fact-sheets/detail/physical-activity

[7] International Diabetes Federation (IDF). Published for World Diabetes Day, IDF Diabetes Atlas. 2021. Available from: www.diabetesatlas.org

[8] M. Kamdem Tienoue Guillaume. Connaissances et attitudes pratiques des diabétiques sur l'activité physique, Thèse présentée Pour obtenir le grade de Docteur en Médecine (Diplôme d'Etat), Faculté de Médecine de Pharmacie et D'Odonto-Stomatologie, Université de Bamako. 2010. Available from: https://www.keneya.net/fmpos/theses/2010/med/pdf/10M255.pdf

[9] Louis Monnier, Claude Colette. Diabétologie, Diabète et activité physique, 3ème édition, Elsevier Masson, ISBN: 9782294758898| EISBN: 9782294759451. 2019. Available from: https://www.elsevier.com/fr-fr/connect/medecine/diabete-et-activite-physique

[10] Mohammad R. The effect of moderate-intensity sports physical activity on blood sugar level and body weight. Sports Creativity Journal. 2020;**11**(2):191-206

[11] Salama BE-DI. Biochemical Characteristics of Sports Physiology, Dar Al-Fikr Al-Arabi. 1st ed2007

[12] Mendelson M, Guinot M, Favre-Juvin A, Wuyam B, Flore P. Aspects méthodologiques de la mesure du lipoxmax : conditions d'application pour les personnes atteintes de pathologies métaboliques. Movement & Sport Sciences. 2014;**84**:61-70

[13] Achten J, Gleeson M, Jeukendrup AE. Determination of the exercise intensity that elicits maximal fat oxidation. Medicine and Science in Sports and Exercice. 2002;**34**(1):92-97

[14] World Health Organization. Body mass index-BMI, Genève. 2020. Available from: https://www.euro.who.int/en/health-topics/disease-prevention/nutrition/a-healthy-lifestyle/body-mass-index-bmi

[15] Zerf M. Effects of walking training performed using continuous and interval

methods on weight loss as effective strategies among postpartum women. Baltic Journal of Health and Physical Activity. 2019;**11**(1):54-61

[16] Groop LC, Eriksson J, Ekstrand A, Franssila-Kallunki A, Saloranta C, Miettinen A. Metabolic characteristics of autoimmune diabetes mellitus in adults, Springer Link. Diabetologia. 1991;**34**:46-51

[17] Chang HK. The Effects of 15 Weeks Walking Exercise Intervention on Physical Fitness and Blood Biochemical Values among Obese Elementary School Students, Department of Leisure and Recreation Management; Chao, Che-Yi; Chao-Chien. 2012. pp. 15-16-17

Chapter 5

Obesity Center and Weight Control

Mahcube Cubukcu and Nur Simsek Yurt

Abstract

Obesity is a multifactorial disease resulting from the complex interaction of genetic, metabolic, behavioral, and environmental factors. Obesity centers, which provide a multidisciplinary approach, play an important role in the implementation of appropriate and sustainable obesity management. The primary objective of obesity centers is to help individuals develop healthy lifestyle skills, achieve, and maintain their target weight, and change their environmental and social habits.

Keywords: obesity, obesity center, body mass index, weight control, treatment

1. Introduction

The World Health Organization (WHO) defines obesity as the abnormal and excessive accumulation of fat in the body to such an extent that it may present a risk to and impair human health [1]. Body mass index (BMI), calculated as body weight in kilograms divided by the square of height in meters, is a simple index commonly used to classify overweight and obesity. For adults, current guidelines issued by the United States Center for Disease Control and Prevention (CDC) and WHO define a normal BMI range as 18.5–24.9, indicating BMI $\geq$25 kg/m^2 as overweight, BMI $\geq$30 kg/m^2 as obesity, and BMI $\geq$40 kg/m^2 as severe obesity [1, 2]. According to this simple definition, obesity is a multifactorial disease that results from a chronic positive energy balance, i.e., when dietary energy intake exceeds energy expenditure. It results from the complex interaction of multiple genetic, metabolic, behavioral, and environmental factors, which are thought to be the primary reasons for the significant increase in the prevalence of obesity [3, 4]. Excess energy is converted into triglycerides, which are stored in adipose tissue, which expands, increasing body fat and causing weight gain. The globalization of food systems, which encourages passive overconsumption of more processed and affordable foods and energy-dense, nutrient-poor foods and beverages, has been identified as a major contributor to the epidemic of obesity [5]. Reduced physical activity associated with modernized lifestyles is also a significant factor [6, 7].

2. The prevalence of obesity

Obesity can occur at any age. Previous studies assessing trends in obesity have reported that the prevalence of obesity is increasing in both adults and children of all ages, regardless of geographic region, ethnicity, or socioeconomic status [8]. In low-income countries, obesity is particularly prevalent among middle-aged adults (especially women) from wealthy and urban backgrounds, whereas in high-income countries it affects both sexes and all age groups [5]. The global prevalence of overweight and obesity has doubled since 1980, with around a third of the world's population now classified as overweight or obese [8]. According to the World Health Organization's 2019 data, Turkey is the 17th most obese country in the world, with 32.1% of the population in Turkey scoring a BMI above 30 [1]. The increasing prevalence of obesity not only affects individuals but also places a significant burden on healthcare systems. In the USA, the healthcare costs incurred by a single obese individual were estimated at USD 1901 per year in 2014, with a national estimate of USD 149.4 billion [9]. The total direct and indirect costs attributable to overweight and obesity in Europe are equivalent to 0.47–0.61% of gross domestic product (GDP) [10].

3. Approach to treatment of obesity

Obesity, which has evolved into a major public health problem affecting physical and mental health, is the second leading cause of preventable death after smoking [11]. Approximately 3 million people die from obesity every year [12]. Obesity is a risk factor for a wide range of medical conditions, including type 2 diabetes, some types of cancer, cardiovascular diseases, and musculoskeletal disorders [12–14]. In addition to these health risks, adverse effects on quality of life and impaired quality of life have been reported to be associated with the degree of obesity [15]. Obese patients have an elevated risk of body image disturbance, low self-esteem, depression, and anxiety [16, 17]. Obese patients cannot lose weight effectively because they do not make diet and exercise indispensable habits of their lifestyles, and even if they manage to lose weight, they cannot maintain their weight. Throughout this long process, patients have a greater chance of success thanks to a multidisciplinary team [18].

Lifestyle intervention and weight loss programs for adults often report disappointing results and diminishing effectiveness associated with low participation and compliance rates [19]. Obese people have been demonstrated to adopt inhibited attitudes toward behavioral change [20]. Therefore, the implementation of lifestyle changes necessary to achieve treatment goals can be extremely challenging [19].

One of the most common behavioral strategies used in weight loss interventions is to help patients identify barriers to behavior change and generate solutions [21]. Perri et al. defined a problem-solving model that recommends active problem-solving for everyday problems for obese people and reported that people who completed problem-solving training lost more weight in the long term [22]. In addition to studies reporting that patients with improved or enhanced problem-solving skills are more likely to adhere to treatment and lose weight, recent meta-analysis reports show that such interventions have significant effects on session attendance and physical activity [19, 23].

Treatment of obesity can be planned according to the clinical characteristics of the patient and may include diet, exercise, medical and surgical treatment [2]. For the diagnosis and assessment of obesity in clinical practice, new approaches have been proposed [3, 4, 24]. Although BMI is commonly used to assess and classify obesity, it has not been proven to be an accurate tool for identifying complications associated with adiposity [4]. Waist circumference is independently associated with increased cardiovascular risk but is not a strong indicator of visceral adipose tissue on an individual basis [25]. Incorporating both BMI and waist circumference into the clinical assessment may identify a higher-risk phenotype. In addition to BMI and waist circumference measurements, a thorough history, appropriate physical examination, and relevant laboratory investigations to identify the root causes of obesity will help identify those who will benefit from treatment [26].

4. Obesity centers and weight control

Obesity centers have been in operation in Turkey to implement appropriate and sustainable obesity management and to treat obese patients using a multidisciplinary approach model [27]. These centers are mission-driven centers that help people who are overweight or obese to reach and maintain their ideal weight [7, 28, 29]. Patients with a BMI of 30 kg/m^2 and above are admitted to obesity centers. Obesity centers have experienced teams that offer a holistic approach to patients. These teams include doctors, dieticians, physiotherapists, psychologists, and nurses [17, 18].

Age, sex, educational level, social and marital status, reading culture, work and adaptation to the center, economic status, residential and daily life status data, attendance at the center, and additional disease information of the patients applying to the obesity center are being collected and recorded. Laboratory tests include complete blood cell count parameters, fasting plasma glucose (FPG), electrolytes, kidney and liver function tests, high-density lipoprotein cholesterol (HDL-C), low-density lipoprotein cholesterol (LDL-C), triglycerides (TG), total cholesterol (TC), and thyroid function tests. Patients receive a total of twelve training sessions at the center at least 3 days a week during the first month, a total of at least six sessions during the second month, and a total of at least three sessions during the third month. Patients who are required to attend training sessions will be categorized according to whether they attend these sessions. Patients who do not attend half of the twelve training sessions during the first month, those who do not attend half of at least six training sessions during the second month, and those who do not attend at least one of the three training sessions during the third month are considered as not attending training [29]. Individualized diet and exercise programs and a medical approach under the supervision of a doctor are planned to achieve the target weight. The aim is to ensure that people who have reached their target weight maintain their healthy lifestyle and weight, change their environmental and social habits, and maintain their weight permanently. If the target weight is lower than the weight to be lost, the program is repeated and the target weight is reset and the time to start losing weight again is planned [28]. Studies have revealed that patients who regularly attend obesity centers lose weight more easily and exhibit significant improvements in serum lipid parameters [29].

Author details

Mahcube Cubukcu[1]* and Nur Simsek Yurt[2]

1 Department of Family Medicine, Samsun University Faculty of Medicine, Samsun, Turkey

2 Clinic of Family Medicine, Samsun Training and Research Hospital, Samsun, Turkey

*Address all correspondence to: mahcube@gmail.com

References

[1] Obesity and overweight. Available from: https://www.who.int/news-room/fact-sheets/detail/obesity-and-overweight [Accesed: September 17, 2023]

[2] The society of endocrinology and metabolism of Turkey. 2019. Available from: https://file.temd.org.tr/Uploads/publications/guides/documents/20190506163904-2019tbl_kilavuz5ccdcb9e5d.pdf?a=1 [Accesed: August 13, 2023]

[3] Mechanick JI, Hurley DL, Garvey WT. Adiposity-based chronic disease as a new diagnostic term: The American Association of Clinical Endocrinologists and American College of endocrinology position statement. Endocrine Practice. 2017;**23**(3):372-378

[4] Garvey WT, Mechanick JI. Proposal for a scientifically correct and medically actionable disease classification system (ICD) for obesity. Obesity (Silver Spring). 2020;**28**(3):484-492

[5] Swinburn BA, Sacks G, Hall KD, McPherson K, Finegood DT, Moodie ML, et al. The global obesity pandemic: Shaped by global drivers and local environments. Lancet. 2011;**378**(9793):804-814

[6] Ladabaum U, Mannalithara A, Myer PA, Singh G. Obesity, abdominal obesity, physical activity, and caloric intake in US adults: 1988 to 2010. The American Journal of Medicine. 2014;**127**(8):717-27 e12

[7] Karatepe EO, Cubukcu M, Simsek YN. Evaluation of the level of physical activity and quality of life in patients registered to the obesity center: Samsun province example. The Journal of Kırıkkale University Faculty of Medicine. 2023;**25**(2):248-259

[8] Network GBoDC. Global Burden of Disease Study 2017 (GBD 2017) Results. Seattle, United States: Institute for Health Metrics and Evaluation (IHME); 2018

[9] Kim DD, Basu A. Estimating the medical care costs of obesity in the United States: Systematic review, meta-analysis, and empirical analysis. Value in Health. 2016;**19**(5):602-613

[10] Von Lengerke T, Krauth C. Economic costs of adult obesity: A review of recent European studies with a focus on subgroup-specific costs. Maturitas. 2011;**69**(3):220-229

[11] Cubukcu M, Ture E, Yazıcıoğlu YE. The relationship of vitamin d status with body mass index among obese patients registered to the obesity center. Türkiye Aile Hekimliği Dergisi. 2021;**25**(2):47-52

[12] Tobias DK, Hu FB. The association between BMI and mortality: Implications for obesity prevention. The Lancet Diabetes & Endocrinology. 2018;**6**(12):916-917

[13] Guh DP, Zhang W, Bansback N, Amarsi Z, Birmingham CL, Anis AH. The incidence of co-morbidities related to obesity and overweight: A systematic review and meta-analysis. BMC Public Health. 2009;**9**:88

[14] Anandacoomarasamy A, Caterson I, Sambrook P, Fransen M, March L. The impact of obesity on the musculoskeletal system. International Journal of Obesity. 2008;**32**(2):211-222

[15] Kolotkin RL, Andersen JR. A systematic review of reviews: Exploring

the relationship between obesity, weight loss and health-related quality of life. Clinical Obesity. 2017;7(5):273-289

[16] KavehFarsani Z, Kelishadi R, Beshlideh K. Study of the effect of family communication and function, and satisfaction with body image, on psychological well-being of obese girls: The mediating role of self-esteem and depression. Child and Adolescent Psychiatry and Mental Health. 2020;**14**:39

[17] Balkoca F, Cubukcu M, Simsek YN. The relationship between obesity with depression and anxiety levels: A cross-sectional, case-control study. Turkish Journal of Diabetes and Obesity. 2023;7(2):152-158

[18] Belibagli MC, Celikkanat S. Problem-solving self-appraisals of obese patients. European Review for Medical and Pharmacological Sciences. 2019;**23**(23):10498-10500

[19] Burgess E, Hassmen P, Welvaert M, Pumpa KL. Behavioural treatment strategies improve adherence to lifestyle intervention programmes in adults with obesity: A systematic review and meta-analysis. Clinical Obesity. 2017;7(2):105-114

[20] Mauro M, Taylor V, Wharton S, Sharma AM. Barriers to obesity treatment. European Journal of Internal Medicine. 2008;**19**(3):173-180

[21] Nezu CM, Nezu AM, Colosimo MM. Case formulation and the therapeutic alliance in contemporary problem-solving therapy (PST). Journal of Clinical Psychology. 2015;**71**(5):428-438

[22] Perri MG, Nezu AM, McKelvey WF, Shermer RL, Renjilian DA, Viegener BJ. Relapse prevention training and problem-solving therapy in the long-term management of obesity. Journal of Consulting and Clinical Psychology. 2001;**69**(4):722-726

[23] Fitzpatrick SL, Wischenka D, Appelhans BM, Pbert L, Wang M, Wilson DK, et al. An evidence-based guide for obesity treatment in primary care. The American Journal of Medicine. 2016;**129**(1):115.e1-115.e7

[24] Sharma AM. M, M, M & M: A mnemonic for assessing obesity. Obesity Reviews. 2010;**11**(11):808-809

[25] Grundy SM, Neeland IJ, Turer AT, Vega GL. Waist circumference as measure of abdominal fat compartments. Journal of Obesity. 2013;**2013**:1-9

[26] Hruby A, Hu FB. The epidemiology of obesity: A big picture. PharmacoEconomics. 2015;**33**(7):673-689

[27] Circular on the opening, registration, working procedures and principles of obesity centers. 2018. Available from: https://shgm.saglik.gov.tr/TR50203/201829-sayili-obezite-merkezlerinin-acilmasi-tescil-edilmesi-calisma-usul-ve-esaslari-hakkinda-genelgesi.html [Accesed: September 30, 2023]

[28] Obesity centers and obesity surgery applications regulation about. Available from: https://www.resmigazete.gov.tr/eskiler/2023/05/20230506-10.htm [Accesed: September 14, 2023]

[29] Yildirim DI, Eryılmaz MA. Evaluation of patient profile and training effectiveness applying to obesity Center. Ankara Medical Journal. 2020;**20**(2):327-336

Chapter 6

Comparison of BMI Indicators in Participants in Special Olympics and Non-Sporty Children with Intellectual Disability

Jitka Kampasová and Hana Válková

Abstract

The goal of the study is to compare BMI indicators in children who regularly do sports, participating in the Special Olympics (SO) with non-sporty children, show the trend of BMI indicators, and to find out whether the 2-month of summer holidays have any effect on BMI indicators. An InBody device was used. Participants are children and adolescents with intellectual disability (ID). In total, four measurements of children were carried out over the course of 2 years. Total participants SO is n = 14, n = 18, n = 18, and n = 13 (13.6 ± 2.8 aged). Non-sporty children is n = 35, n = 37, n = 38, and n = 46 (12.5 ± 3.1 aged). Participants SO have 1.48 lower BMI values, 1 kg more muscle mass, and 1.3 kg less fat. During the summer holidays, participants SO have an increase in muscle mass (BMI and fat remain unchanged). For non-sporty children, all indicators decrease over the summer holidays (BMI, muscle mass, and fat). Participants SO have better results in all BMI indicators compared to non-sporty children. The results clearly show the great importance of sports and the positive effects of physical activities for children and adolescents with ID.

Keywords: BMI, muscles, fat, SO participants, non-sporty children, InBody, trends

1. Introduction

Overweight and obesity in children are the most significant public health problems and deserve attention in the health care system [1, 2]. Over the past 40 years, the number of obese children and adolescents worldwide has increased 10x (from 11 million to 124 million) [2].

Increased body weight (especially in adolescents) is more common in people with intellectual disability (ID), which is a risk factor for various other diseases [3, 4]. About 47% of adults with ID are obese, and their physical activity levels are insufficient to prevent the disease [5–7].

The situation is similar for children with ID. Children and adolescents with ID are highly prone to obesity, and they often suffer from obesity of the first and second degree [8, 9] and, compared to children without ID, they have far more health problems, which include autism, Down syndrome, epilepsy, cerebral palsy, motor problems, constipation, osteoporosis [10–12], delayed child development, speech problems, and behavioral problems [13].

The risk of overweight and obesity decreases with increasing severity of intellectual disability [14]. In the adult population with ID, women, people with Down syndrome, and people with mild ID have a higher prevalence of obesity [14, 15]. Up to 80% of obese children will be obese as adults [16].

In France, 26% of children with ID are obese and overweight [17]. In Romania, the prevalence of overweight and obesity in adolescents with ID is similar for boys and girls. Twenty-eight percent of boys are obese and 19% of boys are overweight, and 16% of girls are obese and 40% of girls are overweight [18]. In Taiwan, BMI in children and adolescents with ID was found to be related to age, but not to gender, diseases, or prescribed medications. The prevalence of obesity there is 18% [1].

In boys with ID, obesity is associated with early adolescence and with a mild and moderate ID, while in girls, obesity is associated with middle adolescence and with a mild ID [19]. Among the four groups of children, children without ID, children with mild ID, children with severe ID and children with Down syndrome, no statistically significant differences were found in relation to BMI in any category. The BMI of children with ID ranges from 18.5 to 24.9 [20].

When analyzing BMI among Special Olympics (SO) participants from different countries, it was found that participants from the USA have the highest prevalence of obesity who are three times more likely to be obese or overweight compared to participants from other countries [21, 22]. In North America, 30% of children and adolescents who regularly compete in Special Olympics are overweight or obese. The prevalence rate is highest among girls, as 54% of girls are overweight or obese. Increasing age is associated with a higher probability of being overweight and obese. Both age and gender are significant factors for obesity in children with ID [23].

The prevalence of obesity also varies by housing type. Among persons with ID in the USA, the lowest rates of obesity are those living in an institution and the highest rates of obesity are those living in their families [4, 15]. The situation in Europe is similar for children and adolescents with ID. The children who live in the children's home are not obese, but they are normal weight or underweight. Children who live in their own family are obese or normal weight. That is children who live in a children's home have a healthier diet compared to children who live in their family [24].

The level of physical activity is low in children and adolescents with ID [25]. Only half of children with ID have sufficient physical activity [26, 27], which is 12,000 steps per day [28, 29]. At the same time, the positive aspects of sports are therefore far more important for children with ID than for children without disabilities [30, 31]. Physical activity leads to physical and mental health [32], improves aerobic capacity of the lungs, motor skills, and coordination, and also contributes to the visibility and increase of the social status of the person, thereby increasing satisfaction in children and adolescents with ID who regularly do sports [33, 34].

2. Materials and methods

The study took place for 2 years at two elementary schools in the Czech Republic and was part of the nationwide Czech Healthy Community Project, which was financed as part of the Special Olympics by the Golisano Foundation (USA). It is a completely new longitudinal research in BMI indicators in children and adolescents with ID.

BMI indicators were measured at each school a total of four times, each time in June and September, in order to find out if the 2-month summer holiday (July, August) has any effect on children's BMI indicators.

2.1 Goal of the study

The first goal of the study is to compare BMI indicators in children who regularly do sports, participating in the Special Olympics (SO) with non-sporty children.

The second goal of the study is to show the trend of BMI indicators and to find out whether the 2-month summer holidays have any effect on BMI indicators in children.

2.2 Study participants

The study participants are children aged 6–20 years (boys and girls together). In **Table 1**, we see the average age of all participants. SO participants have a mean of 13.6 years and a standard deviation of ±2.8 years, and non-sporty children have a mean of 12.5 years and a standard deviation of ±3.1 years.

The participants are from two elementary schools in the Zlín Region in the Czech Republic. (Both schools cooperate with the Czech Special Olympics Movement). Children have mild or moderate ID. Three children with severe ID were excluded from the study.

The number of SO participants (**Table 2**) was around 18 in each measurement, and the number of non-sporty children was around 40. In total, over 50 children participated in each measurement.

SO participants are children who regularly do sports in the selected sport or sports which are organized by the Czech Special Olympics Movement (ČHSO) in the given region. Sporty children also regularly participate in sports competitions organized by the Czech Special Olympics Movement. Throughout the year, the ČHSO allows

Age	SO Participants		Non-sporty Children	
	Mean	S. deviation	Mean	S. deviation
June 2017	14.3	2.8	12.2	3.2
September 2017	13.7	3.0	12.0	2.8
June 2018	13.3	3.1	13.0	2.9
September 2018	13.3	2.3	12.9	3.5
Average of four measurements	**13.6**	**2.8**	**12.5**	**3.1**

Table 1.
Characteristics of the research group according to the age of the participants.

	June 2017	September 2017	June 2018	September 2018
SO participants	14	18	18	13
Non-sporty children	35	37	38	46
Total	49	55	56	59

Table 2.
Characteristics of the examined group according to the number of participants.

children to play sports and compete both in summer sports, e.g. athletics, swimming, bowling, football, floorball, cycling, etc., and in winter sports, e.g. downhill skiing, cross-country skiing, and snowboarding.

All participants in the study have, as part of the compulsory education at their elementary school, the subject of physical education, which has a time allowance of 2–4 hours per week (children with moderate ID have a higher number of hours of physical education at each school, which is usually in the range of 3–4 hours per week).

2.3 InBody device

The InBody 230 device was used to determine BMI indicators (**Figure 1**). InBody is a very accurate device that has eight touch electrodes and measures the body segment by segment. Using this device, it is possible to determine the exact composition of the body (proportion of muscle mass and body fat), the recommended minimum caloric intake, and energy expenditure in various sports.

BMI or body mass index is defined in kg (a person's weight) per m^2 (the square of a person's height). It was developed as an indicator of disease risk because as BMI increases, so does the risk of certain diseases. With the help of BMI, we can classify every adult into one of the following categories:

- Underweight: under 18.5
- Normal weight: 18.5–24.9

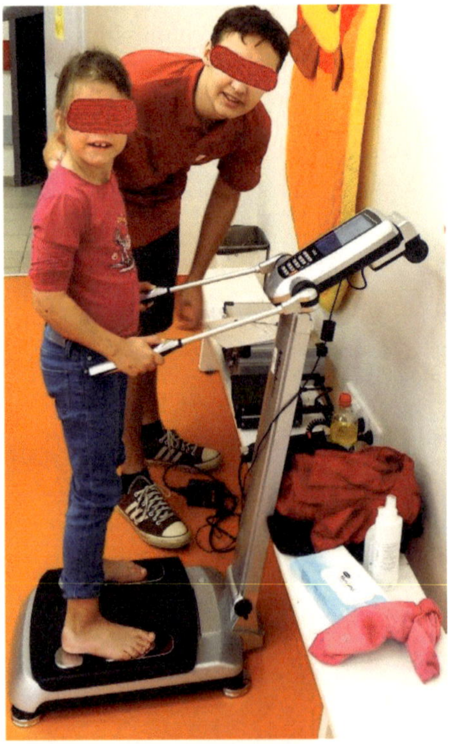

Figure 1.
Measurements on the InBody device.

- Overweight: 25–29.9
- Obesity first degree: 30–34.9
- Obesity second degree: 35–39.9
- Obesity third degree: over 40

BMI is also used in children and adolescents (aged 5–19 years), where the measured BMI value is compared based on the child's gender and age with the Z-score table created by the World Health Organization (WHO), separately for boys and separately for girls. This places the child in one of the following categories: severe underweight, underweight, normal weight, overweight, and obesity [35, 36].

2.4 Project management

Before the start of the study, a personal meeting was held with the principals of the cooperating schools and a Cooperation Agreement was signed with them. Consents for children's participation in the study were then prepared for their parents, and subsequently the consents were distributed to their parents for signature. The study was also approved by the ethics committee of the Faculty of Sports Studies (FSpS) in Brno.

The management of the implementation of the study continued to ensure the dates of the measurements at the schools, to arrange a team of volunteers who went to the schools to help with the measurements and to arrange the borrowing of the InBody device from the FSpS (arranging a single date to suit everyone—it was not easy). As part of the management of the entire project, it was necessary to ensure: uniform T-shirts for volunteers, transport for volunteers, refreshments for all measurement participants (which was a great motivation for the children to participate in the study), and advertising banner with the sponsor's logo. Forms for measurements and other small things (disinfection, writing accessories, tape measure, etc.) were also provided.

Before the actual measurement, the station was being prepared. That is, InBody had to be near an electrical outlet, at another station a meter was placed on the wall to measure the children's height, another station consisted of a table with chairs—the entrance interview with the children took place there, etc.

Measuring children on the InBody was not easy at all, both for the children and for the trained person operating the device (volunteer). It was very difficult for the children to stand still for about 30 seconds on the electrodes of the device and to hold the handles of the device in the given places with their hands. Often the children only measured themselves on the second or third attempt.

2.5 Data analysis

The analysis and evaluation of the data were in program Statistica and Excel. Using normality tests, we found that these are nonparametric data. That is, the data do not fit a Gaussian normal distribution, and therefore, the median (a nonparametric quantity) is presented in the results instead of the arithmetic mean (a parametric quantity that does not fit this data).

Analysis of variance, specifically Friedman's ANOVA, was used to detect statistically significant differences at the 5% significance level (four measurements were

Category	Friedman ANOVA
	p
BMI—SO participants	0.69859
BMI—non-sporty children	0.26948
MUSCLES—SO participants	0.43215
MUSCLES—non-sporty children	**0.01066**
FAT—SO participants	0.29574
FAT—non-sporty children	0.85901

Table 3.
Analysis of variance—Friedman ANOVA.

carried out at each school, on the same group of participants, so these are dependent data). In **Table 3**, we can see that there is a statistically significant difference only between the data in the muscle category in non-sporty children.

Due to the longitudinal research, data analysis (BMI, muscle, and fat) is also carried out in terms of development trends.

3. Results

3.1 Comparison of BMI values in SO participants and non-sporty children

In **Figure 2**, we can see that SO participants have lower BMI values than non-sporty children throughout the research period. Therefore, SO participants have a slimmer figure.

SO participants have a convex trend where they have a different BMI value in each measurement. **Summer holidays therefore have no effect on the BMI value.**

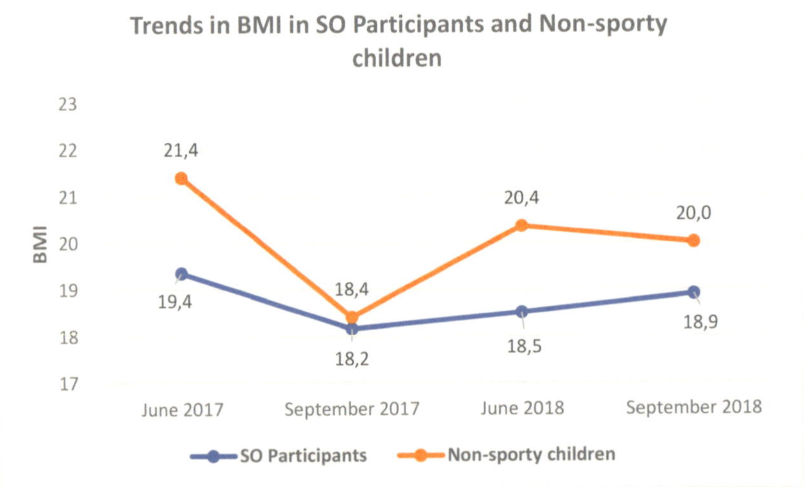

Figure 2.
Comparison of trends in BMI.

DOI: http://dx.doi.org/10.5772/intechopen.107346

BMI	SO Participants				Non-sporty Children				Non-sporty children difference
Median	**S. deviation**	**Min**	**Max**	**Median**	**S. deviation**	**Min**	**Max**	**Compared to SO participants**	
June 2017	**19.35**	4.71	14.30	30.20	**21.40**	25.11	14.10	101.00	**2.05**
September 2017	**18.15**	3.68	13.90	28.70	**18.40**	7.75	12.30	50.40	**0.25**
June 2018	**18.50**	4.79	13.10	32.90	**20.35**	14.44	13.70	101.00	**1.85**
September 2017	**18.90**	4.58	15.20	32.40	**20.00**	13.79	12.90	101.00	**1.10**
Median of four measurements	**18.70**	**4.65**	**14.10**	**31.30**	**20.18**	**14.12**	**13.30**	**101.00**	**1.48**

Table 4.
Descriptive BMI statistics.

Non-sporty children have an unbalanced trend. They always have a lower BMI value in September (in September 2017, they have 18.4 and in September 2018 they have 20), i.e. **summer holidays cause a decrease in BMI.** And this change is not statistically significant (see **Table 3**).

If we compare the children's BMI according to their age (**Table 1**) with the WHO tables created for children (both with the table for boys and with the table for girls), we find that **all participants are in the normal-weight category throughout the research period.**

When comparing the descriptive statistics (**Table 4**), we see a larger range in BMI values for non-sporty children, as the minimum measured BMI values are around 12.30 and the maximum around 101. For SO participants, the minimum BMI values are around 13.10 and the maximum values around 32. Here, we see a big difference in the maximum measured values.

Non-sporty children have a higher BMI value of 0.25 to 2.05. During the entire period of the 2-year research, SO participants have a clearly lower BMI value of 1.48 on average compared to non-sporty children.

3.2 Comparison of MUSCLES values in SO participants and non-sporty children

SO participants have an unbalanced trend (**Figure 3**). They always have a higher muscle value in kg in September (in September 2017, they have 19.5 kg and in September 2018 they have 18.5 kg of muscle), i.e. **summer holidays cause an increase in muscle mass.** And this change is not statistically significant (see **Table 3**).

Non-sporty children have an unbalanced trend. They always have a lower muscle value in kg in September (in September 2017, they have 16.6 kg and in September 2018 they have 18.5 kg of muscle), i.e. **summer holidays cause a loss of muscle mass. And this change is statistically significant** (see **Table 3**).

When comparing the descriptive statistics (**Table 5**), we see that non-sporty children have less muscle by 2 kg (June 2017) and 2.85 kg (September 2017) in the

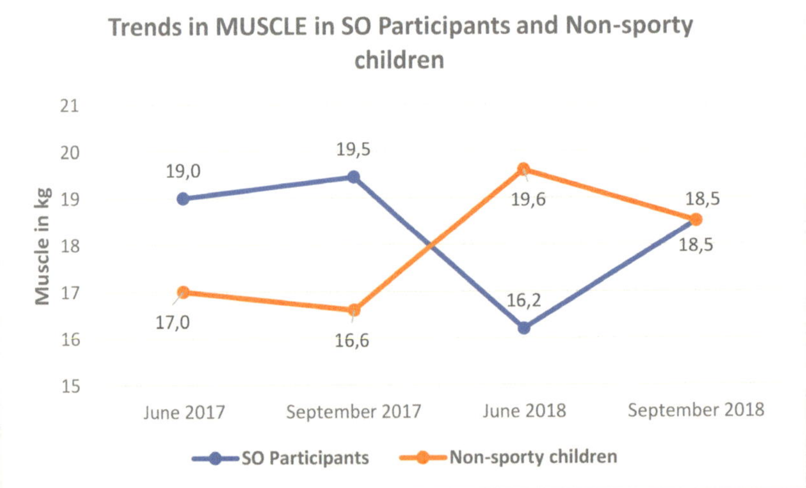

Figure 3.
Comparison of trends in muscle.

DOI: http://dx.doi.org/10.5772/intechopen.107346

Muscles	SO Participants			Non-sporty Children					Non-sporty children difference
Median	**S. deviation**	**Min**	**Max**	**Median**	**S. deviation**	**Min**	**Max**	**Compared to SO participants**	
June 2017	**19.00**	6.70	5.00	29.90	**17.00**	7.26	2.70	34.90	**−2.00**
September 2017	**19.45**	9.04	1.40	42.40	**16.60**	8.29	1.50	42.10	**−2.85**
June 2018	**16.20**	10.55	3.50	44.00	**19.60**	8.02	6.80	46.00	**3.40**
September 2017	**18.50**	5.70	9.30	30.00	**18.50**	8.09	8.20	36.70	**0.00**
Median of four measurements	**18.75**	**7.87**	**4.25**	**36.20**	**17.75**	**8.05**	**4.75**	**39.40**	**−1.00**

Table 5.
Descriptive statistics of muscles in kg.

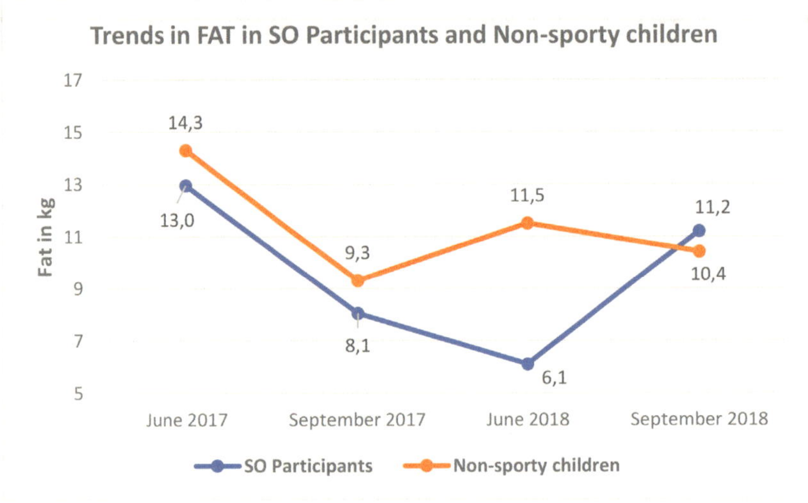

Figure 4.
Comparison of trends in fat.

first two measurements. In the third measurement, non-sporty children have 3.40 kg more muscles, and in the last measurement, both groups have the same amount of muscle.

From the point of view of the measured minimum values and also according to the standard deviation, we see a greater range of muscle mass in sports children. SO participants have on average 1 kg more muscles than non-sporty children.

3.3 Comparison of FAT values in SO participants and non-sporty children

In **Figure 4**, we see that SO participants (blue color) have lower body fat values than non-sporty children in three out of four measurements.

SO participants have a convex trend where they have a different amount of fat in kg at each measurement. **Summer holidays have no effect on body fat.**

Non-sporty children have an unbalanced trend. They always have a lower fat value in kg in September (in September 2017 they have 9.3 kg and in September 2018 they have 10.4 kg of fat), i.e. **summer holidays cause body fat loss**. And this change is not statistically significant (see **Table 3**).

When comparing the descriptive statistics (**Table 6**), we see that non-sporty children have more fat by 1.25 to 5.40 kg in the first three measurements. In the last measurement, non-sporty children have 0.80 kg less fat.

From the point of view of the maximum and minimum values and also according to the standard deviation, we see a greater range of body fat in non-sporty children. SO participants have an average of 1.3 kg less fat than non-sporty children.

4. Discussion

The results clearly show that SO participants have a lower BMI value of 1.48, and they also have 1 kg more muscle and 1.3 kg less fat compared to non-sporty children.

Fat	SO Participants				Non-sporty children				Non-sporty children difference
Median	S. deviation	Min	Max	Median	S. deviation	Min	Max	Compared to SO participants	
June 2017	12.95	8.50	2.60	29.70	14.30	9.95	0.70	43.60	1.35
September 2017	8.05	8.07	1.40	29.90	9.30	15.34	0.60	74.20	1.25
June 2018	6.10	9.00	0.90	34.90	11.50	13.06	1.20	68.00	5.40
September 2017	11.20	8.36	3.00	34.50	10.40	11.72	1.00	47.00	−0.80
Median of four measurements	**9.63**	**8.43**	**2.00**	**32.20**	**10.95**	**12.39**	**0.85**	**57.50**	**1.30**

Table 6.
Descriptive statistics of fat in kg.

Sports and physical activity are therefore important factors for children with ID in shaping their body composition. A number of authors agree on the positive effects of sport for children with ID, but they describe the effects of sport rather generally, i.e. that sport in children leads to physical and psychological health [32], to the improvement of functional indicators such as increasing the aerobic capacity of the lungs, lowering the heart rate, and lowering the blood pressure. Furthermore, as a result of adaptation to physical stress, tendons become stronger, muscles grow, and bones become stronger. In the psychological field, sport leads to an increase in self-confidence, visibility, and higher subjective satisfaction of a person [33, 34, 37]. It is also proven that regular exercise has an effect on daily life in children with ID—on the area of self-care, i.e. progress was found in food, clothing, personal hygiene, and also communication [38].

For non-sporty children, their BMI values decrease during the summer holidays. It follows that during the summer holidays (when children do not have to sit in school desks for several hours every day), children have much more physical activities, which have a positive effect on their body composition. At the same time, it seems that the children only engage in spontaneous movement and not targeted sports activities, because their muscle mass and amount of fat decrease during the summer holidays. (Regular physical activity would be a prerequisite for an increase in muscle mass in children).

Both SO participants and non-sporty children are in the normal-weight category according to BMI throughout the 2-year research period. Czech children are not obese. Obesity is agreed upon by a number of foreign authors, according to which roughly 20–50% of children with ID have obesity [8, 9, 18, 21, 22].

In the Czech Republic (ČR), the school system for children with ID is well set up, as even non-sporty children are in the normal-weight category. The 2 to 4 hours of physical education per week that all children have at school is therefore sufficient for them. The whole range of activities that teachers and children engage in throughout the school year is also important. Part of the regular education includes, for example, self-service training, preparation of simple meals, various school trips during the year, music therapy, snoezelen (a specially designed room to support the perception of all the senses contains, for example, a water cylinder, starry sky, water bed, aroma lamp, etc., to calm down and reduce stress and tension), canistherapy, basal stimulation, etc. Another important factor is that only trained teachers who understand their work can work in schools in the ČR, and children therefore have professional teaching in all subjects.

5. Conclusions

SO participants have a convex trend in BMI, with summer holiday having no effect on their BMI. Non-sporty children have an unbalanced trend in BMI, and summer holidays cause their BMI values to decrease. During the entire period of the 2-year research, SO participants have a clearly lower BMI value of 1.48 on average compared to non-sporty children.

SO participants have an unbalanced trend in their muscles, and the summer holidays cause an increase in their muscle mass. Non-sporty children also have an unbalanced trend in their muscles, and summer holidays cause a decrease in their muscle mass, and this change is statistically significant. SO participants have on average 1 kg more muscles than non-sporty children.

SO participants have a convex trend in fat, with summer holiday having no effect on their fat. Non-sporty children have an unbalanced fat trend, and summer holidays cause their body fat to decrease. SO participants have an average of 1.3 kg less fat than non-sporty children.

Overall, children with ID in the Czech Republic have very good results in BMI indicators, as both sports and non-sporty children have a normal weight. Czech children have much better results in BMI indicators than children abroad.

The results clearly show the great importance of sports and physical activities for children with ID, as well as the well-established school system in the Czech Republic and its cooperation with the Czech Special Olympics Movement, which enables children to do sports all year round. The current trend of education and the Czech Special Olympics Movement should be maintained in the future.

Author details

Jitka Kampasová* and Hana Válková
Faculty of Sports Studies of Masaryk University, Department of Social Sciences and Sport Management, Brno, Czech Republic

*Address all correspondence to: jitka198@seznam.cz

References

[1] Lin JD, Yen CF, Li CW, Wu JL. Patterns of obesity among children and adolescents with intellectual disabilities in Taiwan. Journal of Applied Research in Intellectual Disabilities. 2005;**18**(2):123-129. DOI: 10.1111/j.1468-3148.2005.00241.x

[2] NCD Risk Factor Collaboration. Worldwide trends in body-mass index, underweight, overweight, and obesity from 1975 to 2016: A pooled analysis of 2416 population-based measurement studies in 128·9 million children, adolescents, and adults. Lancet. 2017;**390**:2627-2642. DOI: 10.1016/S0140-6736(17)32129-3

[3] Melville CA, Hamilton S, Hankey CR, Miller S, Boyle S. The prevalence and determinations of obesity in adults with intellectual disabilities. Obesity Reviews. 2007;**8**(3):223-230. DOI: 10.1111/j.1467-789X.2006.00296.x

[4] Rimmer JH, Yamaki K. Obesity and intellectual disability. Mental Retardation and Developmental Disability Research Reviews. 2006;**12**(1):70-82. DOI: 10.1002/mrdd.20091

[5] Forman-Hoffman VL, Ault KL, Anderson WL, Weiner JM, Stevens A, Campbell VA, et al. Disability status, mortality, and leading causes of death in the United States community population. Medical Care. 2015;**53**(4):346-354. DOI: 10.1097/MLR.0000000000000321

[6] Froehlich-Grobe K, Lee J, Washburn RA. Disparities in obesity and related conditions among Americans with disabilities. American Journal of Preventive Medicine. 2013;**45**(1):83-90. DOI: 10.1016/j.amepre.2013.02.021

[7] Yu S, Wang T, Zhong T, Qian Y, Qi J. Barriers and facilitators of physical activity participation among children and adolescents with intellectual disabilities: A scoping review. Healthcare Basel. 2022;**10**(2):233. DOI: 10.3390/healthcare10020233

[8] Heryati E, Ratnengsih E. Adaptive physical education model for increasing physical fitness of children with intellectual disability. Advances in Social Science Education and Humanities Research. 2017;**118**:202-207

[9] Salaun L, Berthouze-Aranda SE. Physical fitness and fatness in adolescents with intellectual disabilities. Journal of Applied Research in Intellectual Disabilities. 2012;**25**(3):231-239. DOI: 10.1111/j.1468-3148.2012.00659.x

[10] Aljerf L, Aljurf M. Improvements in the ecological and nutritional aspects of down's syndrome. Preprint 2020. 2020. DOI: 10.21203/rs.3.rs-30313/v1

[11] Oeseburg B, Dijkstra GJ, Groothoff JW, Reijneveld SA, Jansen DE. Prevalence of chronic health conditions in children with intellectual disability: A systematic literature review. Intellectual and Developmental Disabilities. 2011;**49**(2):59-85. DOI: 10.1352/1934-9556-49.2.59

[12] Tyler CV, Schramm S, Karafa M, Tang AS, Jain A. Electronic health record analysis of the primary care of adults with intellectual and other developmental disabilities. Journal of Policy and Practice in Intellectual Disabilities. 2010;**3**:204-210. DOI: 10.1111/j.1741-1130.2010.00266.x

[13] Emerson E, Brigham P. The developmental health of children of parents with intellectual disabilities: Cross sectional study. Research in Developmental Disabilities.

2014;**35**(4):917-921. DOI: 10.1016/j.ridd.2014.01.006

[14] Melville CA, Cooper SA, Morrison J, Allan L, Smiley E, Williamson A. The prevalence and determinants of obesity in adults with intellectual disabilities. Journal of Applied Research in Intellectual Disabilities. 2008;**21**(5):425-437. DOI: 10.1111/j.1468-3148.2007.00412.x

[15] Stancliffe RJ, Lakin KC, Larson S, Engler J, Bershadsky J, Taub S, et al. Overweight and obesity among adults with intellectual disabilities who use intellectual disability/developmental disability services in 20 US States. American Journal on Intellectual snd Developmental Disabilities. 2012;**116**(6):401-418. DOI: 10.1352/1944-7558-116.6.401

[16] Wiklund P. The role of physical activity and exercise in obesity and weight management: Time for critical appraisal. Journal of Sport and Health Science. 2016;**5**(2):151-154. DOI: 10.1016/j.jshs.2016.04.001

[17] Salaun L, Berthouze-Aranda S. Obesity in school children with intellectual disabilities in France. Journal of Applied Research in Intellectual Disabilities. 2011;**24**(4):333-340. DOI: 10.1111/j.1468-3148.2010.00612.x

[18] Ungurean BC, Cojocariu A, Abalasei BA, Popescu L, Puni AR, Stoica M, et al. The analysis of the correlations between BMI and body composition among children with and without intellectual disability. Children-Basel. 2022;**9**(5):582. DOI: 10.3390/children9050582

[19] Králíková J, Válková H. BMI indicators in children with intellectual disabilities. Studia Sportiva. 2019a;**13**(1):85-97. DOI: 10.5817/StS2019-1-9

[20] Ungurean BC, Cojocariu A, Puni AR, Oprean A. Body mass index in children with and without intellectual disability: Distribution and implications. Proceedings of the 6th International Conference of Universitaria Consortium FEFSTIM: Physical Education, Sports and Kinesiotherapy - Implications in Quality of Life. 2020. pp. 331-335

[21] Harris N, Rosenberg A, Jangda S, O'Brien K, Gallagher ML. Prevalence of obesity in International Special Olympic athletes as determined by body mass index. Journal of the American Dietetic Association. 2003;**103**(2):235-237. DOI: 10.1053/jada.2003.50025

[22] Li H, Frey GC, McCormick BP, Johnston JD. Comparison of obesity among Chinese and US Special Olympic athletes with intellectual disabilities. Research in Developmental Disabilities. 2015;**41**:94-100. DOI: 10.1016/j.ridd.2015.05.005

[23] Lloyd M, Temple VA, Foley JT. International BMI comparison of children and youth with intellectual disabilities participating in Special Olympics. Research in Developmental Disabilities. 2012;**33**(6):1708-1714. DOI: 10.1016/j.ridd.2012.04.014

[24] Králíková J, Válková H. Trends in body mass index among children with mild and moderate intellectual disabilities. Studia Sportiva. 2019b;**13**(2):42-54. DOI: 10.5817/StS2019-2-5

[25] Cho C, Shin W, Kong S. Participation in regular physical activity according to the type of disability, sex, point of disability diagnosis, and ability to walk independently in South Korea. Healthcare Basel. 2021;**9**(8):1079. DOI: 10.3390/healthcare9081079

[26] Shields N, Dodd KJ, Abblitt C. Do children with down syndrome perform

sufficient physical activity to maintain good health? A pilot study. Adapted Physical Activity Quarterly. 2009;**26**(4):307-320. DOI: 10.1123/apaq.26.4.307

[27] Wouters M, Evenhuis HM, Hilgenkamp TIM. Physical activity levels of children and adolescents with moderate-to-severe intellectual disability. Journal of Applied Research in Intellectual Disabilities. 2019;**32**(1): 131-142. DOI: 10.1111/jar.12515

[28] Colley RC, Jansen IAN, Tremblay MS. Daily step target to measure adherence to physical activity guidelines in children. Medicine and Science in Sports and Exercise. 2012;**44**(5):977-982. DOI: 10.1249/MSS.0b013e31823f23b1

[29] WHO. Global recommendations on physical activity for health. Geneva, Switzerland: WHO; 2010b

[30] Dykens EM, Rosner BA, Butterbaugh G. Exercise and sports in children and adolescents with developmental disabilities - Positive physical and psychosocial effects. Child and Adolescent Psychiatric Clinics of North America. 1998;7(4):757. DOI: 10.1016/S1056-4993(18)30210-4

[31] Zull A, Tillmann V, Froboese I, Anneken V. Physical activity of children and youth with disabilities and the effect on participation in meaningful leisure-time activities. Cogent Social Sciences. 2019;**5**(1). DOI: 10.1080/23311886.2019.1648176

[32] Kapsal NJ, Dicke T, Morin AJS, Vasconcellos D, Maiano C, Lee J, et al. Effects of physical activity on the physical and psychosocial health of youth with intellectual disabilities: A systematic review and meta-analysis. Journal of Physical Activity & Health. 2019;**16**(12):1187-1195. DOI: 10.1123/jpah.2018-0675

[33] Johnson CC. The benefits of physical activity for youth with developmental disabilities: A systematic review. American Journal of Health Promotion. 2009;**23**(3):57-167. DOI: 10.4278/ajhp.070930103

[34] Lahtinen U, Rintala P, Malin A. Physical performance of individuals with intellectual disability: A 30-year follow-up. Adapted Physical Activity Quarterly. 2007;**24**(2):125-143. DOI: 10.1123/apaq.24.2.125

[35] WHO. A healthy lifestyle - WHO recommendations. 2010a. Retrieved from: http://www.euro.who.int/en/health-topics/disease-prevention/nutrition/a-healthy-lifestyle/body-mass-index-bmi (see 27 July, 2022)

[36] WHO. BMI for age 5-19. 2007. Retrieved from: https://www.who.int/toolkits/growth-reference-data-for-5to19-years/indicators/bmi-for-age (see 27 July, 2022)

[37] Jančík, J., Závodná, E., Novotná, M. Fyziologie tělesné zátěže-vybrané kapitoly. Brno: Masarykova Univerzita. 2006. Retrieved from: https://is.muni.cz/elportal/estud/fsps/js07/fyzio/texty/index.html (see 29 July, 2022)

[38] Chadwick OB, Cuddy M, Kussel Y, Taylor E. Handicaps and the development of skills between childhood and early adolescence in young people with severe intellectual disabilities. Journal of Intellectual Disability Research. 2005;**49**(12):877-888. DOI: doi.org/10.1111/j.1365-2788.2005.00716.x

Chapter 7

Weight Loss through Aquatic Exercise

Fariba Hossein Abadi

Abstract

Obesity is one of the main causes of unwanted health-related issues. Obese people have a more limited ability to keep fit although they are seriously willing to do exercise and improve their physical fitness. While there are numerous methods and programs to reduce weight through land-based exercises, there still exist reluctance, discomfort and risks of injury during exercise for obese people. However, an effective exercise program should plan at a moderate intensity level with low-perceived exertion for obese people. Then aquatic exercise can be purposed as a convenience exercise without joint strain and high impact. Considering the physical properties of water, aquatic aerobic exercise not only can increase metabolic demand and burn calories but immersing the body in water provides a non-weight bearing exercise option. Consequently, the relevant knowledge about aquatic exercise assists to provide proper exercise programming as well as consideration of physical fitness programs for obese who are unwilling to do land-based exercise. As a background of obesity prevalence is presented in this chapter, there are focuses on aquatic exercise definition and its benefits as well the exercise prescription for weight loss. Then, a perspective of aquatic exercise for obese people and concise guidelines are reviewed in this chapter.

Keywords: aquatic exercise, weight loss, obesity, obese people, aqua exercise prescription

1. Introduction

This chapter will explain weight loss through aquatic exercise. This section focuses on a concise of obesity prevalence, aquatic exercise definition, and its benefits for obese people. Besides that, this chapter will explain the aquatic exercise prescription designed for weight loss, as well. Hence, this chapter creates an opportunity to extend the superiority of aquatic aerobic exercise as a convenient and effective exercise training method to lose weight and improve physical fitness components, which led to the reduction of the health risk factors for different overweight and obese groups.

1.1 Obesity definition and BMI

Obesity is commonly defined as having great body mass. Then, Body Mass Index (BMI) is a term that is mostly applied to determine the weight in link to stature or height.

Basically, BMI is particularly computed as an individual's weight in kilograms divided by the square of height in meters which shows via $kg{\cdot}m^{-2}$ unit. Commonly, the American College of Sports Medicine (ACSM) guidelines define the overweight class as a BMI of ≥25, the obese class as a BMI of ≥30 $kg.m^{-2}$, and the extremely obese class as a BMI of ≥40 $kg.m^{-2}$ [1], while Suissa et al., based on WHO report in 2020, have displayed the different BMI values for adult men and women across the globe [2]. In this regard, there are different BMI values for different countries worldwide, for example in South East Asia BMI of ≥28 $kg.m^{-2}$ is defined as obesity class. In addition, another accurate definition by WHO [3] considers abdominal obesity through a waist-to-hip ratio (WHR) which in men is more than 0.90 and for women, it's a ratio of 0.81 or more.

1.2 Obesity prevalence

In general, overweight and obesity are caused by additional accumulated fat in adipose tissues which is the main cause of unwanted health-related issues. It is approximately half a century (since 1975) that obesity has almost tripled globally. Alam, and Agrawal [4] stated according to WHO report [5], more than 1.9 billion adults in the age of 18 years and older, were categorized as overweight class, while 650 million of those were in the obese class (BMI ≥30 $kg.m^{-2}$) [4]. In addition, right before the COVID-19 pandemic (in 2019), it was estimated that 38.2 million children (<5 years old) were in the classes of overweight or obese. Even though previously overweight and obese were tabled as a problem in the high-income country, currently being overweight and obese are on the rise in low- and middle-income countries, specifically in urban settings [6]. However, the evidence displayed since 2000, the number of overweight children (<5 years old) has augmented by nearly 24% in Africa. Approximately half of these overweight or obese children (<5 years old) were in 2019 and lived in Asian countries. In 2020, also, there were 39 million children (<5 years old) were classified as overweight or obese. Meanwhile, Afshin et al., in the study entitled "Health effects of overweight and obesity in 195 countries over 25 year" stated the World Health Organization estimated that till 2018, 39% of adults were overweight and 13% of them were obese in the world. They also stated in 2015, there were overall 107.7 million obese children and 603.7 million obese adults, which is expected to rise in the future [7].

Nowadays, it is well-documented that obesity is a complicated health problem and it is outcomes from contributing several factors, such as genetics, individual behaviors (e.g., physical activity and dietary habits), the cultural and community environment. It also can be the result of the effect of disease or medications. In other words, physical inactivity, daily anxiety stressors, increasing sitting time and unhealthy food intake result in overweight and obesity. However, the rate of sitting time and sedentary lifestyle most likely will lead to obesity which indirectly can affect dramatically on cardiorespiratory health [8].

However, excess fat impairs the organs and body systems function, leading to multiple health problems and even decease. Heart disease, diabetes, hypertension, hypertriglyceridemia and some forms of cancers are altogether related to obesity and can be fatal. Meanwhile, other health disparities conditions such as low-back pain, osteoarthritis, sleep disorder, psychological impairments, and reproductive issues are also common although not life-threatening. Then, overweight and obese people need to access superior knowledge to manage their weight to an ideal and healthy condition. However, obese people need to do lifestyle modification and significantly target three key components including a healthy diet, regular exercise, as well as behavior therapy [1].

Hence, to avoid the epidemic of high cardiovascular risk conditions and the relevant diseases, such as obesity, diabetes, and hypertension people must change their sedentary lifestyles toward a physically active lifestyle. In that, engaging in physical activities such as aerobic exercise programs have been a popular choice among the obese community. Then, obese people are required to improve their health and fitness and nowadays in modern life which is more vital and valuable during their young ages.

However, metabolic demands can greatly rise during and after exercise. It is obvious these increases result in superior caloric expenditure which is highly dependent primarily on the type of exercise. On this point, particularly aquatic aerobic exercise as a convenience, non-weight bearing exercise for individuals who are obese or overweight can be recommended as a significant intervention program not only for weight loss but for the betterment of cardiovascular fitness also.

2. Aquatic exercise program for obese people

Although several research studies were directed to reduce weight and enhance well-being through exercise programs carried out on land, there still exist difficulty, discomfort and risks of injury when performing programmed exercise for obese people. Besides, the obese population has also shown reluctance to exercise due to being ashamed of their body feature.

It should be considered that the exercise programs are challenging due to the limited ability of obese people to perform the exercise more effectively without joint strain, high impact, injury risk, and the overall discomfort associated with land exercise [9]. Then, water-based exercises are also highly beneficial to overweight or obese individuals.

Meanwhile, previous studies suggested that an exercise program with moderate intensity levels and low perceived exertion should be proposed for the obese as an effective exercise program, particularly for obese people with poor mood status and low self-efficacy. Therefore, water-based exercises are a suitable alternative form of exercise for the overweight and obese population. The following sections focus on aquatic exercises and their benefits for obese people.

2.1 What is aquatic exercise?

The aquatic exercise consists of an exercise program that is performed in water. According to Aquatic Exercise Association, water-based exercise or aquatic exercise programs were first developed by the National Arthritis Foundation YMCA [10], for therapeutic medium and health care services [11]. In the past four decades, a variety of specific aquatic exercises have developed to achieve rehabilitation and fitness purposes for people with difficulty in physical exercise on land. In addition, several studies verified aquatic exercise not only can enhance the health-related fitness components including cardiovascular fitness, muscle strength and muscle endurance, flexibility and balance, but it can decrease quickly the body fat percentage of obese patients with arthritis and also among disabled population and elder people. It has also a significant multiple health outcomes and positive physical and psychological effects [11]. Moreover, an aquatic exercise program which is also entitled water aerobics, aqua aerobics, shallow or deep-water walking/jogging/running or aqua biking/spinning exercise, or similar heading names. It is reported that they are safer than land-based exercise to decrease the risk of injuries and difficulty of exercising [12].

All types of the aquatic exercises require water-immersed and typically are performed as aerobic exercises in shallow water media like a swimming pool. The aquatic exercise is mostly performed vertically, without swimming strokes skills and typically in waist-deep, chest-deep or deeper water a type of resistance training.

However, any apparent restrictions like obesity, low levels of physical fitness, locomotion difficulties caused by aging, and some disabilities, or diseases can limit the ability of people to exercise [13]. In that, due to this limitation, aquatic exercises can be offered as a suitable alternative compared to land-based exercises.

2.2 Relevant terms for aquatic exercise

Aquatic exercise as an alternative exercise program is also called:

Water exercise programs, Water-based exercise, Aqua/water aerobics, Shallow or Deep water walking/running exercise, Aqua aerobic exercise, Water-based exercise, Aqua fitness, Aqua Yoga, Aqua Zumba, Aqua cycling, Aqua spinning and so on [1].

3. Benefits of aquatic exercise for obese people

There are several advantages of aquatic exercise for the obese population including the following:

- High energy demanding (easy to burn calories)
- Improved cardiovascular stamina
- Increases vital energy
- Low impact exercise; weightless (Perceived rate of exertion is less)
- Lessens of the gravity effect
- Lessens heart disease risk factors
- Hydrostatic pressure to assist venous return
- Easier to adhere to do exercise (due to cool media, comfortable, relaxing and hidden the fatness and body shape)
- Great place to start water walking (Xiphoid depth)
- Self-selected speed
- Emphasize safety
- Provide relaxation; feel weightless
- Less fear of falling or injuring self in the water
- Mental aspects of water; reduces anxiety, depression, ...

3.1 Aquatic exercise and energy expenditure

Physical properties of water allow it to be a valuable tool in physical conditioning and exercise. The density of water is determined nearly 800 times of air. Then, workout in the water media provides high level of demanding and expending energy with less essential effort to the body to burn calories in order to losing weight [9]. Furthermore, numerous studies have examined the impact of different aqua aerobic exercises on obesity and cardiovascular risk factors. They revealed the significant heightening in health advantage in elderly people similar to aerobic exercise on land [14, 15]. A previous study conducting a program of aquatic exercise (12 weeks, 3 days weekly, 70 minutes) showed significant enhancement in cardiorespiratory fitness. The study also revealed a decrease in body fat percentage (8% reduction in skin-fold thickness), an increase in peak VO_2 (12%), muscular strength, and a diminish in total cholesterol in older-adult women [16].

Furthermore, several types of research clearly indicated that obese people are effectively able to expend energy or burn calories in a vertical position of aquatic workouts. It seems that the resistance of the water makes up for the reduced workload associated while there is non-weight bearing in the buoyant media [1]. The most effective variables that increase the burning calories as energy expenditure during aquatic exercise in vertical immersion in the water include the following:

- Depth of water that effect on weight bearing, movement control, and the resistance quantity.
- Movement speed that acts on the quantity of dragging propulsion and resistance.
- Amount of force which act against the water resistance (e.g., workout intensity; more calories you burn if the work is harder).
- Length of the individual limbs, which affects the amount of resistance which encountered during moving against the water.
- Environmental aspects such as water temperature of water and air, humidity and chemicals.

Table 1 Shows the comparison of energy expenditure of the exercising in the land-based versus the water-based exercise. The energy expenditure estimated for 30 minutes workout for a person with 70 kg with xiphoid level of immersion (tolerate of 25% of total weight).

Land-based (calories)	Water- based (calories)
Walking: 102	Walking: 220
Jogging: 230	Jogging: 340
Aerobic: 175	Aerobic: 240

Table 1.
Comparing energy expenditure of aerobic activities on land vs. water (estimation for a person with 70 kg and 30 minutes workout).

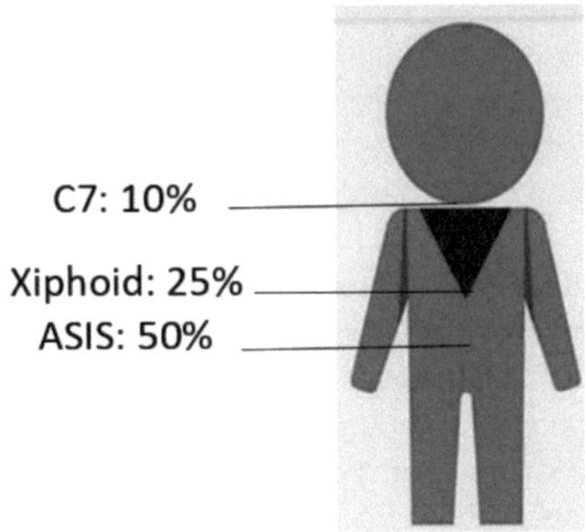

Figure 1.
Depth of water immersion and weight bearing.

3.2 Depth of immersion on weight bearing

There are numerous studies that investigated the influence of body immersion levels and the intensity of aquatic exercises. Firstly, the rate of perceived exertion (RPE; 0–10 scale; exercise intensity) is higher at the hip level immersion compared to immersion up to the chest. The increased scale of RPE may be due to the higher intensity of drag forces acting in the lower limbs, as compared to those acting in the trunk and upper limbs when partially immersed. Secondly, shallow water reduces the buoyancy and increases ground reaction force and then the changes in the neuromuscular pattern of active muscles at different levels of the body in the water.

When comparing shallow-water versus deep-water exercises, the physiological demand seems to be lower for deep-water exercises which are helpful for individuals. In total immersion position, weight-bearing is affected by the water depth owing to buoyancy as well. As **Figure 1**. shows, in general, weight-bearing is depending on water immersion level which determined at the seventh cervical vertebral level (C7), the xyphoid, and the anterior superior iliac (ASIS) approximately 10, 25, and 50% of their body weight, respectively [12].

Then, decreasing depth of water is one way to progress lower extremity weight bearing. However, the depth of immersion can reflect static weight bearing, and effect on the speed of movement like fast or slow walking or running in water. In that, exercising in water makes feel about 90% lighter while viscosity of water creates a resistance exercise atmosphere. In another words, this condition makes water exercise, with low impact, an ideal activity for obese people. In summary, aquatic aerobic exercise will increase energy expenditure while the body immersing in water and weigh up to 90% (neck-line) less than on land and it is non-weight bearing nature [12]. Meanwhile, although a few aquatic studies reported there was no improvement in weight loss, those planned appropriate aquatic exercise programs (e.g., frequency, duration, intensity and study length) have clearly resulted in weight loss [1].

4. Precautions and contraindications

In spite of aquatic exercise program can effortlessly assist to lose weight, and improve quality of life among obese population, many obese still have limitation and difficulty to join the aquatic exercise. Therefore, while the advantages of aquatic exercise are considerable, the potential risks also should be determined to create appropriateness of aquatic exercise program. In that, the policies and procedures should be specified basis of the precautions and contraindications [1, 12]. Some of the special precautions and contraindications include the following:

- Fear of water (water phobia)
- Neurologic disorders
- Uncontrolled Seizures
- Cardiac/respiratory dysfunction
- All infections and open wounds
- Contagious skin rashes
- Kidney disease (inability of urine output)
- Chlorine or bromine allergy
- Unstable blood pressure
- Uncontrollable bowel/bladder
- Non-tunnel catheters
- Epilepsy (problems with glare)
- Aspiration
- Severe impulsivity
- The danger of bleeding or hemorrhage

4.1 Warning signs

It is important to monitor the obese individual either during exercise time, or while they relax at a normal water temperature. It is not only essential to start the aquatic exercise program with 50–55% of intensity, but the below warning signs are always considerable during each session:

- Light-headedness
- Nausea
- Headache
- Dizziness

- Increased pain
- Agitation
- High fever

5. Aquatic exercise as fitness and weight loss program

While a variety of physical activity and exercise program has provided health and weight management program, in the past four decades, aquatic exercise training became an alternative and favorable program for fitness and rehabilitation purpose for obese or people who have physical difficulty exercising on the ground [9]. In addition, proper breathing technique consists of controlling time of inhale, exhale, and holding breath during exercising significantly improve the capability of cardiorespiratory fitness (CRF) and some cardio metabolic biomarker [17]. While the risk of cardiovascular disease increases progressively when blood pressure (BP) indicates above 115/75 mmHg [18] among obese people, water-based exercise is as an effective method of physical activities and exercise to decrease stress and high blood pressure [19, 20].

Typically, water applies as a resistance for similar exercises that normally are done on land, such as jogging or jumping jack. It is mostly performed with individuals who are not skilled in swimming strokes. Additionally, aquatic exercise offers equal benefits as other types of exercise, but it provides a lower risk of injuries to the muscles and joints while recovering cardiorespiratory fitness, muscular fitness, body composition, agility, flexibility, and also blood lipids in obese populations and older adults [12].

Besides, water-based exercise, also called aqua aerobics, aqua exercise, aquatic dance exercise, water workouts, or hydro aerobics, is an activity that can leave participants feeling exhilarated. Water exercise often performed to music, provides a workout for the heart and lungs, as well strengthening and toning muscles [11]. It is obvious that being free from the effects of gravity makes movement easier in water. Interestingly, anyone can have fun in a water exercise class. Individuals do not have to be able to swim and do not need previous experience to achieve success. Some aquatic classes use music during the workout. Obese participants in water aerobics classes (at least 30 minutes) can effortlessly burn about 300 calories. Many workouts in the aquatic classes include stretching exercises, kicking, jumping, squats, dance movements and warm-ups, a cool-down or relaxation period.

Aquatic aerobics exercise is commonly more low-impact than land-based exercises, while participants have higher energy expenditure due to the resistance of water. Also, movements tend to perform with slower speed because of the water viscosity.

5.1 Aquatic aerobics exercise programs

Aquatic aerobics exercise, as one of the modern forms of exercise, is becoming more and more popular among the public, specially for obese women. It is a type of resistance training in the water. Aqua aerobic exercise supports the body weight to reduce the risk of injury to the joints and muscles. During stretching the legs in the water, the buoyancy force gives less stress on the joints, which allowed maximum range of motion in water. Aquatic exercise can also improve physical and mental health and overall, the quality of life.

In any aquatic program format, all elements of the program including the needs and abilities of participants, the purpose of the session, the size and shape of the pool, equipment availability, water temperature, and the environment must be considered. According to the American College of Sports Medicine [21] recommendations, the components of training sessions for aquatic exercise are also included a warm-up, conditioning or specific sport-related exercise, and finally stretching and relaxation as a cool-down [1, 11].

Warming-up: An aquatic exercise session warm-up involves a thermal warm-up, pre-stretch, and cardiorespiratory activity continuing at a minimum of 5 minutes. This section will be instructed in a variety and creative ways based on the specific objectives of the aquatic program.

Conditioning phase: in general, the conditioning phase consists of the primary exercise mode such as cardiorespiratory or aerobic training, muscular strength and endurance, stability, flexibility and neuromotor exercise. A conditioning phase in any session can purposively be the combination of these exercise modes.

Cooling-down: Even though, cooling-down can be optional in a session of aquatic exercise, in most aquatic fitness programs, it still consists of two parts including the cardiorespiratory cool-down and the post-stretch. In this part, stretching, deep breathing technique, relaxation movement and self-care and free activity in the water also can usefully be recommended.

5.2 General recommendations

Even though water is a lenient and versatile exercise medium, sometimes older adults, elderly, and obese people will not able to safely perform movements exactly as instructed or intended. Then, the participants' ability, the movement purpose, the class purpose, and the modifications possibility or optional movement should be considered when planning aquatic exercise programs. Using general recommendations for any section of the class and various formats can be attractively designed to keep aquatic classes engaging, provide training variety and motivate obese participants. Therefore, to get started and adhere to aquatic exercise till the ideal weight the following are suggested:

- Exercise with music
- Listen to your body respond
- Take time to conduct periodic assessments
- Record your activities regularly
- If any health problem arises, visit a physician

5.3 Programming considerations

- Safety

Steps, ramps, and ladders may serve as access for safe entry and safe exit at the pool. Participants should be reminded to wear shoes and be aware of clothing to prevent slips or falls and chafing.

- Programming

Exercises that cause discomfort shall be avoided, specifically for those with musculoskeletal considerations, who might need to have an alternative program with low-impact intensity in shallow water. However, to plan an appropriate aquatic exercise program the below factors are considerable:

- Leadership skills
- Suggest the option of wearing aquatic that makes them feel more comfortable.
- Equipment and the knowledge of the usage of each aid-assistant. For example, drag resistance is most suitable for training progression and buoyancy resistance like hand bars may compromise body control.

6. Aquatic exercise guidelines

6.1 Aquatic exercise prescription

According to ACSM [21], a reduction of 3–10 percent of initial weight over 3–6 months by an aerobic exercise program at a moderate intensity level with resistance training is recommended. Then, obese people need to do exercise a minimum of 5 days per week. In other words, the goal of weekly exercise activity should be 300 minutes per week, or approximately 60 minutes per day to burn 500–600 kcal as shown in **Table 2** [1, 7].

6.2 Aquatic exercise intensity

It is essential to monitor aquatic exercise intensity levels to achieve a significant weight loss result. In addition, the ACSM [21] guidelines advise obese people to start aquatic exercise somewhat easily and continue the workout with moderate exercise for a long time. Based upon the Borg Rating of Perceived Exertion (RPE) the Aquatic Exercise Intensity Scale for weight loss purposes is recommended as below:

Start with ~50–55% Aquatic HR: Somewhat easy RPE level. At this intensity level, you feel that you can continue exercising for hours. You can still easily speak in full sentences and have conversations while the breathing and heart rates are slightly increased.

Intensity	Type	Frequency & duration	~kcal	Example of movement
Low to moderate-with resistance	Aerobic interval (1:1 ratio)	3 sessions weekly, 60 minutes	500–600	2 minutes of hard skier jumping jack extension (work): 2 minutes steady wide walk/jogs (recovery)

Table 2.
A summary of aquatic exercise prescription.

Continued with ~60–65% Aquatic HR: Moderate RPE level. At this intensity level, you could do the exercise for a long time. Your breathing and heart rates will noticeably start to rise. Your body is sweating, which reminds you of going beyond a normal exercise level as the muscles feel contractions and start working. Then, at this level, you could continue the activity for a while before having to rest or stop. The proper example to compare this moderate intensity is a brisk walk or like walking up a slight incline. In this condition, you are still able to say four to five words before taking a breath [1].

6.3 Determination of aquatic heart rate

Firstly, stand out of the pool for 3 minutes, and after that determine the heart rate (HR) for 1 minute. Then, similarly, determine a one-minute HR after 3 minutes of standing in the water (submerging at the axillary level of depth). The aquatic HR is determined by subtracting the standing HR in the water from the standing HR out of the water. It should be mentioned that this deduction will be used via the Karvonen formula to determine the target heart rate [1].

However, it is obvious that environmental conditions, medication, caffeine, excessive activity, or unnecessary movement can affect heart rate response once entering the pool. Then, proper supervision should be considered to minimize these factors [11]. However, important factors that influence aquatic exercise Heart Rates (HR) are shown in **Table 3**. In that, carefully applying a proper heart rate is always advisable.

6.4 Immersion level

The buoyancy of the water not only allows it easily to modify high-impact activities, but the immersion in water also reduces the risk of side movements. It also

Factors	Effect
Water temperature	Water is more efficient to cool the body than air. This cooling reduces the impact of heat stress during exercise and allows lowered heart rate response. Then, cooler aquatic media does not allow the heart to work as hard to drive out the produced excess heat during exercise.
Gravity	The water buoyancy lessens the gravity effect on body mass. Bloodstream from extremity limbs assists the heart with less effort, resulting in a lowered heart rate.
Compression	Water acts on all body systems (vascular system) such as compressors and it causes a reduced venous load to the heart than equivalent land-based exercise. In that, the heart with lesser working returns blood from the extremities.
Partial pressure	A molecule of gas under pressure more readily enters a liquid. Oxygen is a gas and blood is a liquid. So, a gas transfer might occur more efficiently due to the pressure of water. This better gas exchange results in a reduction of the requirement of increasing heart rate and bloodstream and finally leads to a lesser workload for the heart.
Hydrostatic pressure and immersion	While an individual horizontally floating (prone or supine position), hydrostatic pressure aids in returning fluid and blood to the heart and lymphatic fluid return. It also makes lower working heart rate and affects respiration (HR is 13–17 bpm on average lower in the water) which consequence in increased vital capacity.
Reduced body mass	Since you weigh less in the water, a reduction in body weight might be partly responsible to have lower aquatic HR.

Table 3.
Influence factors on aquatic heart rates (HR) during exercise.

supports weight for single-limb activities which are too challenging on land. Weight-bearing is affected by the depth of water owing to buoyancy as well. In general, for obese participants, immersion level is recommended on the xiphoid and the anterior superior iliac (ASIS) level with approximately 25% of the body weight [12].

6.5 Water temperature

The water temperature range is suggested to be set between 27 and 30°C (80–86°F) for overweight and obese participants as well as the tempo of the exercise [9].

6.6 Aquatic program formats

- Circuit training:

Circuit training is often an instructor-guided program referred to as station training with any combination and various stations.

- Interval training:

Interval training is implicated in a series of training cycles where the ratio of work–rest sets the basis for training.

- Dance-oriented programs:

The dance-oriented program includes A variety of dance classes with specific styles of dance, like hip-hop, ballet, ballroom, or traditional and ethnic rhythms dances.

- Stride training (Walk and Jog):

Stride training can be designed through striding patterns such as forward and backward walk/jog, and sidewalk/jog. It is also incorporated in different water depths as a warm-up or cool-down format for other aquatic exercise programs also. Walking and jogging training is carried out on treadmill, also.

- Aqua cycle program:

Aqua cycle program or aquatic cycling can be designed with a circuit-training workout or interval training for the improvement of cardiorespiratory fitness. Aquatic cycling can also focus on muscle conditioning also.

- Aqua-step:

An aquatic step program can be set up for the improvement of cardiorespiratory training, muscular fitness, or neuromotor activities. A step (a proper bench or a platform) to step up and down is needed during a class.

- Aqua-pole:

Aqua-Pole exercise format can focus on various health, fitness and rehabilitation protocols. The training program is designed to improve not only overall fitness, but posture, muscular strength, and toning, and also included choreographic techniques to challenge agility, coordination and cardiorespiratory endurance.

- Aqua-trampoline:

Mini trampoline as the elastic nature can offer for unique workout at a low-impact exercise option in water media. In addition, during all movements core muscles need to actively be involved since trampoline surface is unstable.

- Muscular conditioning programs:

This type of training focuses mainly on muscular fitness. It is also offered as a station of a circuit training program for muscle conditioning with specific segments.

- Martial arts programs:

Martial arts–style classes are performed by assigning movement patterns and techniques such as kicks, punches, and blocks into the water. It is carried out with a high-intensity, highly resistive, while it is still an option with a lower-impact exercise [1].

7. Summary

The aquatic exercise program is a non-weight bearing exercise that increases energy expenditure while the body is immersed in water. Aquatic exercise not only can be recommended as a desirable body composition and weight loss for obese people but as an overall health-related fitness component, also. Water-based exercises, specifically aquatic aerobics, can easily help to promote fat loss. As well, the body can build lean tissue or muscle mass while working against the three-dimensional resistance of the water (viscosity). The most effective aquatic exercise program formats for weight loss are comprised of striding (walking/jogging) in shallow or deep depths of water, aquatic step, martial arts style, aquatic dance, aquatic cycling or spinning, and circuit and interval training in shallow water. The training sessions include warm-up, conditioning, stretching and relaxation as a cool-down. The immersion level is mostly recommended on the xiphoid level with approximately 25% of the body weight and the water temperature should be set between 27 and 30°C. For all aquatic exercise programs, obese people should preferably exercise a minimum of 5 days per week for 60 minutes per day at a moderate intensity level with resistance training. Carefully determining aquatic heart rate in order to exercise with an appropriate heart rate and moderate intensity is always advisable. Considering the advantages of aquatic exercise programs, the limitations and potential risks for obese people also should be determined and all special precautions and contraindications need to be thought out.

Author details

Fariba Hossein Abadi
Faculty of Sports Science and Coaching, Department of Health Science, Sultan Idris Education University (UPSI), Tanjong Malim, Perak, Malaysia

*Address all correspondence to: fariba@fsskj.upsi.edu.my

References

[1] Aquatic Exercise Association. Aquatic Fitness Professional Manual. 7th ed. Champaign, Illinois: Human Kinetics; 2018

[2] Suissa K et al. Validation of obesity-related diagnosis codes in claims data. Journal of Diabetes, Obesity. 2021;**23**(12):2623-2631

[3] World Health Organization. World health statistics 2020. 2020

[4] Alam I, Agrawal S. Introduction to obesity. In: Obesity, Bariatric and Metabolic Surgery: A Practical Guide. Springer; 2016. pp. 3-11

[5] World Health Organization. World health statistics 2023: Monitoring health for the SDGs, sustainable development goals. World Health Organization; 2023

[6] Haththotuwa RN et al. Worldwide Epidemic of Obesity, in Obesity and Obstetrics. Elsevier; 2020. pp. 3-8

[7] Afshin A et al. Health effects of overweight and obesity in 195 countries over 25 years. New England Journal of Medicine. 2017;**377**(1):13-27

[8] Huxley R et al. Body mass index, waist circumference and waist: Hip ratio as predictors of cardiovascular risk – A review of the literature. European Journal of Clinical Nutrition. 2010;**64**(1):16-22

[9] Abadi HF et al. Effects of aqua-aerobic exercise on the cardiovascular fitness and weight loss among obese students. International Journal of Physiotherapy. 2017;**4**(5):278-283

[10] Boutaugh ML, Brady TJ. Quality of life programs of the Arthritis Foundation. Orthopaedic Nursing. 1996;**15**(5):59-73

[11] Aquatic Exercise Association. Standards and Guidelines for Aquatic Fitness Programming: The Global Resource in Aquatic Fitness. Nokomis, FL.; 2008. pp. 2-4. Retrieved December 18, 2008

[12] Abadi HF et al. A perspective on water properties and aquatic exercise for older adults. International Journal of Aging Health Movement. 2020;**2**(2):1-10

[13] Abadi FH et al. The effect of aquatic exercise program on low-back pain disability in obese women. Journal of Exercise Rehabilitation. 2019;**15**(6):855-860. DOI: 10.12965/jer.1938688.344

[14] Scheer A et al. Twelve weeks of water-based circuit training exercise improves fitness, body fat and leg strength in people with stable coronary heart disease: A randomised trial. Journal of Physiotherapy. 2021;**67**(4):284-290. DOI: 10.1016/j.jphys.2021.08.012

[15] Stan EA. The benefits of aerobic aquatic gymnastics on overweight children. Palestrica of the Third Millennium Civilization & Sport. 2012;**13**(1):27-30

[16] Takeshima N et al. Water-based exercise improves health-related aspects of fitness in older women. Medicine & Science in Sports & Exercise. 2002;**34**(3):544-551

[17] Jasiński R et al. Effect of nordic walking and water aerobics training on body composition and the blood flow in lower extremities in elderly women. Journal of Human Kinetics. 2015;**45**(1):113-122

[18] Delevatti R, Marson E, Kruel LF. Effect of aquatic exercise training on lipids profile and glycaemia: A systematic

review. Revista Andaluza de Medicina del Deporte. 2015;**8**(4):163-170

[19] Kim SB, O'sullivan DM. Effects of aqua aerobic therapy exercise for older adults on muscular strength, agility and balance to prevent falling during gait. Journal of Physical Therapy Science. 2013;**25**(8):923-927

[20] Piotrowska-Calka E. Effects of A 24-week deep water aerobic training program on cardiovascular fitness. Biology of Sport. 2010;**27**:95-98

[21] Riebe D, Ehrman JK, Liguori G, Magal M, American College of Sports Medicine. ACSM's guidelines for exercise testing and prescription. Lippincott Williams & Wilkins; 2018